MW01482902

Stepping Stones to Living Well with Dysphagia

Nestlé Nutrition Institute Workshop Series

Vol. 72

Stepping Stones to Living Well with Dysphagia

Editors

Julie Cichero Brisbane, Australia

Pere Clavé Barcelona, Spain

KARGER

Nestlé Nutrition Institute

Nestec Ltd., 55 Avenue Nestlé, CH–1800 Vevey (Switzerland)
S. Karger AG, P.O. Box, CH–4009 Basel (Switzerland) www.karger.com

Library of Congress Cataloging-in-Publication Data

Nestlé Nutrition Workshop (72nd : 2012 : Barcelona, Spain)
  Stepping stones to living well with dysphagia / editors, Julie Cichero,
Pere Clavé.
       p. ; cm. -- (Nestlé Nutrition Institute workshop series, ISSN
1664-2147 ; v. 72)
  Includes bibliographical references and index.
  ISBN 978-3-318-02113-4 (hard cover : alk. paper) -- ISBN 978-3-318-02114-1
(e-ISBN)
  I. Cichero, Julie A. Y. II. Clavé, Pere. III. Nestlé Nutrition Institute.
IV. Title. V. Series: Nestlé Nutrition Institute workshop series ; v. 72.
1664-2147
  [DNLM: 1. Deglutition Disorders--Congresses. W1 NE228D v.72 2012 / WI
250]

  616.3'23--dc23
                                           2012029498

The material contained in this volume was submitted as previously unpublished material, except in the instances in which credit has been given to the source from which some of the illustrative material was derived.
    Great care has been taken to maintain the accuracy of the information contained in the volume. However, neither Nestec Ltd. nor S. Karger AG can be held responsible for errors or for any consequences arising from the use of the information contained herein.

Printed on acid-free and non-aging paper
ISBN 978-3-318-02113-4
e-ISBN 978-3-318-02114-1
ISSN 1664-2147
e-ISSN 1664-2155

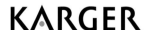

KARGER   Basel · Freiburg · Paris · London · New York · New Delhi · Bangkok ·
            Beijing · Tokyo · Kuala Lumpur · Singapore · Sydney

Contents

For more information on related publications, please consult the NNI website: www.nestlenutrition–institute.org

Preface

Oropharyngeal dysphagia is a major complaint among many patients with neurological diseases and in the elderly. Oropharyngeal dysphagia is specifically classified by the World Health Organization in the International Statistical Classification of Diseases and Related Health Problems ICD-9 and ICD-10 (787.2, R13). The severity of oropharyngeal dysphagia varies from moderate difficulty to complete inability to swallow, and may give rise to clinically relevant complications such as aspiration pneumonia, malnutrition and/or dehydration, impaired quality of life and death. There is a big discrepancy between the high prevalence, morbidity, mortality and costs caused by nutritional and respiratory complications of oropharyngeal dysphagia and the low level of resources dedicated to dysphagic patients.

The main aim of the Second International Course on Oropharyngeal Dysphagia, the 72nd Nestlé Nutrition Institute Workshop 'Stepping Stones to Living Well with Dysphagia' held at the Hospital de Mataró, Spain, May 5–6, 2011, was to educate on science-based state-of-the-art practices in dysphagia patient care to improve the clinical management of our patients with oropharyngeal dysphagia. Our aim was to give the attendants five messages about oropharyngeal dysphagia to take home: (a) oropharyngeal dysphagia is a very frequent and serious symptom with specific nutritional and respiratory complications that can lead to death; (b) dysphagia can be diagnosed, and we provided them clinical methods for screening and complementary explorations for accurate diagnosis; (c) dysphagia can be treated, and treatment is cost-effective because complications are avoided; (d) diagnosis and treatment of dysphagia require a multidisciplinary approach involving several professional domains and interdisciplinary dysphagia care, and (e) research into new strategies is required to understand the pathophysiology and new treatments for impaired swallow response.

Over the two days of the course, we heard top dysphagia specialists from around the world present and discuss the state-of-the-art of science-based methods of diagnosis, treatment and dysphagia patient care. In addition, several practical sessions with real patients, discussion of clinical cases and practices with products provided the participants with real examples of application of all this knowledge in a real clinical setting. The program of the course was also designed to promote networking, communication and interaction within attendants and speakers. This publication promoted by the Nestlé Nutrition Institute includes some of the most relevant presentations of the course, and the conclusions provide a short summary and conclusions of the discussions and deliberations during the meeting.

We believe that identification of oropharyngeal dysphagia as a major neurological and geriatric syndrome will cause many changes in the provision of medical and social services in the near future. Education of health care professionals in diagnosis and treatment of dysphagia and its complications, early diagnosis, development of specific complementary explorations in the clinical setting, improvement in therapeutic strategies to avoid aspirations and malnutrition, and research into its pathophysiology are the cornerstones to allow maximal recovery potential for patients with functional oropharyngeal dysphagia. This book represents an excellent starting point for this process.

Julie Cichero
Pere Clavé

Foreword

Epidemiologic studies suggest that 22% of individuals over 50 years suffer from dysphagia, while the prevalence rises to nearly 40% in those over 60 years. Despite its high prevalence, dysphagia is severely underdiagnosed (in 60% of cases) and permitted to go unmanaged (in 66% of cases), even in clinical settings providing specialized care of older adults. Sadly, poorly managed dysphagia is known to diminish patient quality of life and heighten morbidity, mortality, and costs.

Due to the multifactorial etiology and clinical complications associated with dysphagia, the comprehensive needs of patients are best treated by a multidisciplinary health care team. In an effort to spread the use of science-based, state-of-the-art practices in dysphagia, the Nestlé Nutrition Institute organized the 2nd International Course on Oropharyngeal Dysphagia themed 'Stepping Stones to Living Well with Dysphagia', which was also the 72nd in the series of Nestlé Nutrition Institute Workshops. The 2-day theoretical and practical educational event took place at Mataró Hospital in Spain. The program enabled leading clinicians including nurses, speech-language pathologists, dietitians, nutritionists, gastroenterologists, and additional specialties to connect and share best practices with other dysphagia specialists from across the world.

A major success of the course was to bring together a diverse group, from specialists involved in medical practice to those immersed in research including engineers and other scientists. The program stimulated thinking beyond the current approach and inspired consideration of different science-based practices. Participants learned about novel, validated methods that could be applied in daily practice, as well as emerging therapies for dysphagia. All gained skill at a comprehensive set of evidence-based clinical methods for screening, assessing, diagnosing, and identifying the best treatment strategies.

Robust discussion took place. Having a multicultural and multidisciplinary audience made it clear that there are slight differences between countries in dysphagia definitions and in practices. However, the attendees had similar concerns about a shortage of well-organized multidisciplinary teams with well-trained members. Interactive discussions led to a general consensus among participants on the need for further investigation, continued interaction, and greater collaboration. Specifically, the need for developing international standards and patient management protocols that cover several patients groups, rather than having different tools for specific populations. The fact that dysphagia suffers from a lack of recognition by health authorities was a topic of concern for all participants. In order to convince health authorities of the importance of dysphagia, two aspects were proposed as necessary to demonstrate: first, reliable data on the severity of the condition being common among elderly, and second, economic data to demonstrate that the complications associated with dysphagia like malnutrition or aspiration pneumonia considerably increase cost to the healthcare system. All attendees agreed that outcomes would come sooner not by working in isolation, but by working together.

The interest and efforts of many made it possible to take these steps forward as a result of the Workshop. Our thanks go to: the 72nd Nestlé Nutrition Institute Workshop Book Co-Editors, Dr. Julie Cichero from Australia, and Dr. Pere Clavé from Spain, who both exemplify the strong multidisciplinary team collaboration essential for quality dysphagia patient management, as well as the presenters, session facilitators, and attendees, who shared their expertise and perspectives to permit such a rich learning experience.

Prof. Ferdinand Haschke, MD, PhD
Head of
Nestlé Nutrition Institute
Vevey, Switzerland

Dr. Petra Klassen, PhD
Scientific Advisor
Nestlé Nutrition Institute
Vevey, Switzerland

Dr. Kala Kaspar, PhD
Global Medical Affairs Manager
Nestlé Health Science
Vevey, Switzerland

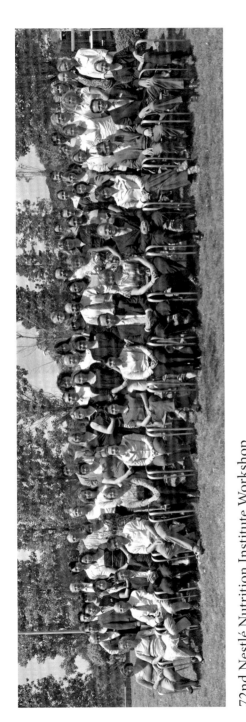

72nd Nestlé Nutrition Institute Workshop

Barcelona, May 5–6, 2011

Contributors

Editors

Dr. Julie Cichero
Honorary Senior Lecturer and Research
Consultant (Speech Pathology)
C/- School of Pharmacy
The University of Queensland
20 Cornwall Street
Brisbane QLD 4102
Australia
E-mail: juliecichero@bigpond.com

Dr. Pere Clavé
Department of Surgery
Hospital de Mataró
Carretera de Cirera s/n
08304 Mataró
Spain
E-mail: pclave@csdm.cat

Speakers & Session Facilitators

Prof. Dr. Jordi Almirall
Intensive Care Unit
Hospital de Mataró
Carretera de Cirera s/n
08304 Mataró
Spain
E-mail: jalmirall@csdm.cat

Dr. Kenneth W. Altman
Mount Sinai School of Medicine
Department of Otolaryngology – HNS
One Gustave L, Levy Place, # 1189
New York, NY 10029
USA
E-mail: kenneth.altman@mountsinai.org

Ms. Patricia Anthony
Head of Medical Affairs
Fresenius Kabi USA
1501 East Woodfield Rd.
Suite 300 East
Schaumburg, IL 60173
USA
E-mail: panthonymd@hotmail.com

Ms. Viridiana Arreola
Hospital de Mataró
Carretera de Cirera s/n
08304 Mataró
Spain
E-mail: viriarreola@gmail.com

Ms. Mireia Arus Figa
Hospital de Mataró
Carretera de Cirera s/n
08304 Mataró
Spain
E-mail: mireiaarus@hotmail.com

Mr. Didier Bleeckx
Grand Hôpital de Charleroi
Grand Rue, 3
6000 Charleroi
Belgium
E-mail: didier.bleeckx@ghdc.be

Dr. Margareta Bülow
Diagnostic Centre of Imaging and
Functional Medicine
Skåne University Hospital
Södra Förstadsgatan 101
SE 205 02 Malmö
Sweden
E-mail: margareta.bulow@med.lu.se

Dr. Rosa Burgos Peláez
Nutritional Support Unit
University Hospital Vall d'Hebron
Pg Vall d'Hebron 119-129
08830 Barcelona
Spain
E-mail: rburgos@vhebron.net

Ms. Anna Ciurana
Hospital de Mataró
Carretera de Cirera s/n
08304 Mataró
Spain
E-mail: aciurana@csdm.es

Dr. Alfonso Cruz-Jentoft
Servicio de Geriatría
Hospital Universitario Ramón y Cajal
Ctra.Colmenar, km 9,1
28034 Madrid
Spain
E-mail: acruz.hrc@salud.madrid.org

Dr. Roberto Dantas
Departamento de Clinica Médica
Faculdade de Medicina de Ribeirão Preto
Universidade de São Paulo
Av. Bandeirantes 3900
14049-900 Ribeirão Preto SP
Brazil
E-mail: rodantas@fmrp.usp.br

Dr. Daniele Farneti
Audiology and Phoniatrician Unit
ENT Divisione, OspedaleInfermi
Via Settembrini 2
47900 Rimini
Italy
E-mail: dfarneti@auslrn.net

Dr. Shaheen Hamdy
School of Translational Medicine –
Epithelial Sciences
Faculty of Medical and Human Sciences
University of Manchester
Clinical Sciences Building
Salford Royal Hospital
Eccles Old Road
M6 8HD, Salford
UK
E-mail: shaheen.hamdy@manchester.
ac.uk

Dr. Kala Kaspar
Global Medical Affairs
Nestlé Health Science
55, Avenue Nestlé, B.P. 353
1800 Vevey
Switzerland
E-mail: kala.kaspar@nestle.com

Dr. Rosemary Martino
Department of Speech Language
Pathology
University of Toronto
160-500 University Ave.
Toronto, ON M5G 1V7
Canada
E-mail: rosemary.martino@utoronto.ca

Ms. Rosa Monteis
Hospital de Mataró
Carretera de Cirera s/n
08304 Mataró
Spain
E-mail: rmonteis@csdm.cat

Dr. Jose Nart
Nart Dental Clinic
Padilla 368
08025 Barcelona
Spain
E-mail: jose@nartperiodoncia.com

Dr. Juan Ochoa
Medical, Scientific, Regulatory Unit
Nestlé Health Sciences
3 Century Drive
Parsipanny, NJ 07054
USA
E-mail: Juan.ochoa@us.nestle.com

Dr. Ernest Palomeras Soler
Hospital de Mataró
Carretera de Cirera s/n
08029 Barcelona
Spain
E-mail: epalomeras@csdm.cat

Ms. Laia Rofes
Laboratori de Fisiologia Digestiva
Hospital de Mataró
Planta -2, porta 64
08304 Mataró
Spain
E-mail: laia.rofes@ciberehd.org

Ms. Marisa Sebastian
Hospital de Mataró
Carretera de Cirera s/n
08304 Mataró
Spain
E-mail: msebastian@csdm.cat

Dr. Renée Speyer
HAN University of Applied Sciences
Institute of Health Studies
Mozartstraat 47
6521 GB Nijmegen
The Netherlands
E-mail: r.speyer@online.nl

Dr. Catriona Steele
Toronto Rehabilitation Institute
550 University Avenue, 12th floor
Toronto, M5G 2A2
Canada
E-mail: catriona.steele@uhn.ca

Dr. Eric Verin
Service de Physiologie
CHU de Rouen
1 rue de Germont
76031 Rouen Cedex
France
E-mail: everin@mac.com

Invited Attendees

Ms. Anne-Sophie Beeckman/Belgium
Ms. Sabrina Delhalle/Belgium
Mr. Luc Van Belle/Belgium
Ms. Teresa Françoise/Brazil
Ms. Brenda Arychuk/Canada
Prof. Zhang Tong/China
Ms. Marylène Ataya/France
Mr. Michel Guatterie/France
Mr. Frédérique Martinet/France
Ms. Patricia Giannika/Greece
Mr. Vasiliki Sideras/Greece
Dr. Hidetaka Wakabayashi/Japan
Ms. Simone Hutten/Netherlands
Ms. Marjan Nijenhuis/Netherlands
Dr. Alexandru Parvan/Romania
Dr. Sonia Abilleira/Spain
Dr. Josep Bassa/Spain
Dr. Eulalia Cabot/Spain
Ms. Esther Cabrera/Spain
Ms. Silvia Carrion/Spain
Dr. Raimundo Gutierriz/Spain
Dr. Omar Ortega/Spain
Mr. Carlos Parra/Spain
Ms. Marisa Pellitero/Spain
Ms. Maria Roca/Spain
Ms. Silvia Zarcero/Spain
Ms. Caroline Lecko/UK

Nestlé HealthCare Nutrition Participants

Mr. Vinciane Szmata/Belgium
Ms. Cindy Steel/Canada
Ms. Zhou Hongyi/China
Mr. Anthony Delhaye/France
Mr. Alessandro Pavone/Italy
Mr. Shinichiro Terasaki/Japan
Ms. Anne Ruizendaal/Netherlands
Mr. Holger Kunze/Singapore
Ms. Carola Granholm/Sweden
Dr. Iva Bogdanova/Switzerland
Ms. Aline Boisset/Switzerland

Dr. Adam Burbidge/Switzerland
Mr. Andreas Busch/Switzerland
Dr. Jan Engmann/Switzerland
Dr. Ivana Jankovic/Switzerland
Prof. Michael Jedwab/Switzerland
Dr. Petra Klassen/Switzerland
Ms. Grainne Mallon/Switzerland

Dr. Simina Popa Nita/Switzerland
Dr. Claire Takizawa/Switzerland
Mr. Remy Charles/UK
Ms. Laetitia Poirier/UK
Ms. Sharan Saduera/UK
Ms. Carol Siegel/USA
Ms. Carrie Tyler/USA

Cichero J, Clavé P (eds): Stepping Stones to Living Well with Dysphagia.
Nestlé Nutr Inst Workshop Ser, vol 72, pp 1–11,
Nestec Ltd., Vevey/S. Karger AG., Basel, © 2012

Definition, Prevalence and Burden of Oropharyngeal Dysphagia: A Serious Problem among Older Adults Worldwide and the Impact on Prognosis and Hospital Resources

Julie A.Y. Cichero[a] · Kenneth W. Altman[b]

[a]School of Pharmacy, The University of Queensland, Brisbane, QLD, Australia; [b]Eugen Grabscheid Voice Center, Department of Otolaryngology – Head and Neck Surgery, Mount Sinai School of Medicine, New York, NY, USA

Abstract

Oropharyngeal dysphagia describes difficulty with eating and drinking. This benign statement does not reflect the personal, social, and economic costs of the condition. Dysphagia has an insidious nature in that it cannot be 'seen' like a hemiplegia or a broken limb. It is often a comorbid condition, most notably of stroke, and many other neurodegenerative disorders. Conservative estimates of annual hospital costs associated with dysphagia run to USD 547 million. Length of stay rises by 1.64 days. The true prevalence of dysphagia is difficult to determine as it has been reported as a function of care setting, disease state and country of investigation. However, extrapolating from the literature, prevalence rises with admission to hospital and affects 55% of those in aged care settings. Consequences of dysphagia include malnutrition, dehydration, aspiration pneumonia and potentially death. The mean cost for an aspiration pneumonia episode of care is USD 17,000, rising with the number of comorbid conditions. Whilst financial costs can be objectively counted, the despair, depression, and social isolation are more difficult to quantify. Both sufferers and their families bear the social and psychological burden of dysphagia. There may be a cost-effective role for screening and early identification of dysphagia, particularly in high-risk populations. Copyright © 2012 Nestec Ltd., Vevey/S. Karger AG, Basel

Introduction

Eating and drinking are essential to human survival as a form of nourishment. Aspects that affect this biological function are naturally a cause for concern.

However, mealtimes also have a social function, and the inability to participate in meals has devastating consequences including depression and social isolation for those affected and their significant others. The act of eating and swallowing requires intact cortical function, oral intake and manipulation, tongue propulsion allied with pharyngeal squeeze and larynx elevation, laryngeal closure with cricopharyngeal relaxation, and proper esophageal function. Of these five components, oropharyngeal function is pivotal to aspiration protection. While there are many possible etiologies and comorbidities, dysphagia is associated with prolonged hospitalization and higher risk of mortality in some populations. In order to adequately discuss the prevalence and burden of oropharyngeal dysphagia in older adults, it is first necessary to clarify our subject matter.

Definitions

Interest in dysphagia has built steadily over the last 30 years. At its most general, *dysphagia* is defined as 'difficulty moving food from the mouth to the stomach' [1]. On the other hand, *deglutition* is generally given to describe the preparatory, oral, pharyngeal and esophageal phases of swallowing [2]. This latter description paves the way for clarification of oropharyngeal versus esophageal dysphagia. Oropharyngeal dysphagia encompasses the oral preparatory, oral and pharyngeal phases of swallowing. The oral preparatory phase includes difficulties associated with biting, closure of the lips, chewing and mastication, mixing of the bolus with saliva, and segmenting the bolus in the oral cavity for safe swallowing. It is under voluntary control. The oral phase includes the ability to contain and control the bolus. The tongue provides the bolus with shaping, transport through and propulsion into the pharynx; this is also part of the oral phase. The pharyngeal phase consists of transport of the bolus through and removal of residue from the pharynx. Once the bolus has passed through the upper esophageal sphincter, the pharyngeal phase has been completed and the esophageal phase has commenced. Both the pharyngeal and esophageal phases are reflexive. The esophageal phase involves bolus transport through the esophagus and into the stomach. Impairments in the esophageal phase may be the consequence of obstruction or motility issues. This information is summarized in figure 1.

While the traditional description of deglutition involves the phases listed above, the brain (cortex and brainstem) plays important roles in the cognition and reflexes involved in swallowing. Also, the role of the larynx should not be excluded, as intact sensation, true and false vocal fold closure and cricopharyngeal relaxation are supremely important.

This paper will focus on the prevalence and burden of *oropharyngeal* dysphagia utilizing the description above. The consequences of oropharyngeal dysphagia broadly affect (1) respiratory safety (aspiration), and (2) swallowing

Cichero · Altman

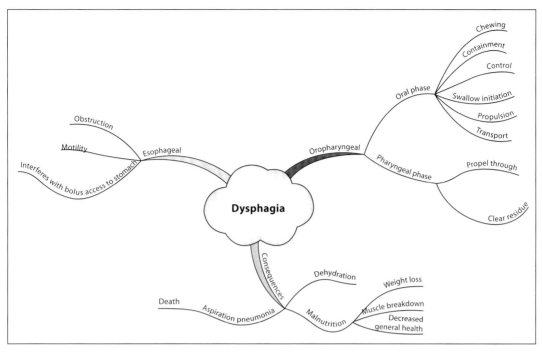

Fig. 1. Definition: oropharyngeal dysphagia vs. esophageal dysphagia.

efficiency (adequacy of nutrition and hydration per oral route). The consequences of oropharyngeal dysphagia will be discussed in detail in other papers in this volume.

The World Health Organization describes 'older adults' as those individuals who are over 60 years of age, and in developed countries, those over 65 years of age. In the popular press, older adults are usually classified as those who have reached retirement age. This varies from country to country. For example, in Australia the retirement age is 65 years, whilst in Norway it is 67 years. In the research literature, older adults are classified as those over 70 years, with a mean age of 84 years [3]. In other literature, 85 years of age is classified as 'the oldest old' [4]. In the study by Cabre et al. [3], older adults with dysphagia presenting to acute care were most likely to:
- Have a poor functional capacity
- Have a geriatric diagnosis (e.g. previous stroke, dementia)
- Live in a nursing home
- Take a large number of medications
- Take a larger proportion of medications that affect level of consciousness or affect the swallowing response (e.g. sedatives, antipsychotic medications, antidepressants)

Prevalence of Oropharyngeal Dysphagia

The true prevalence of oropharyngeal dysphagia is difficult to determine. Research studies have categorized prevalence according to disease state (e.g. stroke); setting (e.g. acute hospital, nursing home, community dwelling) and country of interest. Due to differences in culture, lifestyle habits, diet, health care services and practices, and data collection processes, the ability to generalize findings from one country to another is difficult [5]. Naturally, the prevalence fluctuates according to each of these variables. In the acute care setting, the prevalence ranges from 0.35% physician recorded [6] to 25% assessed [7], and as high as 55% of elderly individuals consecutively admitted to hospital with pneumonia (Spain) [3]. Altman et al. [6] utilized data from a large hospital survey database. In the latter studies with very high prevalence rates, dysphagia screening tools were used to identify individuals at risk of dysphagia and/or aspiration. In the nursing home setting, the figures are more pronounced with prevalence rates between 55 (USA study) [8] and 68% (Canadian study) [9]. Those dwelling in the community show a different prevalence picture. Oropharyngeal dysphagia prevalence figures of 11, 13 and 16% have been reported in the UK, Japan and the Netherlands, respectively, for older community-dwelling residents [10–12]. It should be noted that in the acute and nursing home settings, diagnosis of oropharyngeal dysphagia was confirmed by formal dysphagia assessment. However, community prevalence data come from self-reports on questionnaires. It is likely that the community prevalence of oropharyngeal dysphagia is higher than that formally documented in the research literature.

In 2002, a study conducted over four European countries examined the social and psychological impact of dysphagia [13]. The investigators found that of the group sampled, only 40% reported receiving a formal diagnosis of dysphagia. Country to country variation in symptoms was noted. For example, nursing home residents in the UK and Spain were more likely to report difficulties swallowing thin liquids, whilst individuals in Germany and France were less likely to report these difficulties. Individuals in the UK and France had the highest percentage of coexisting medical conditions (79 and 81%), compared with those residents in Germany and Spain (43 and 67%). A third of all residents in the study needed personal assistance when eating.

Prevalence data for oropharyngeal dysphagia have also been presented according to disease state. Stroke is the condition most commonly linked with dysphagia with a wide prevalence of between 14 and 94% [14]. However, other conditions that affect the central nervous system also present with risk for dysphagia. For example, dysphagia has been reported in one third of individuals with Parkinson's disease [15], and by the time of death reports of up to 81% prevalence of dysphagia have been reported in individuals with motor neuron disease [16].

The prevalence of oropharyngeal dysphagia increases with advancing age. 10–30% of individuals older than 65 years are estimated to have swallowing difficulties [17]. Increasing age is associated with increased risk for dysphagia. The prevalence of other comorbidities, such as stroke, also increases with advancing age; hence, age risks are most likely associated with comorbidity risks. Individuals aged over 65 years represented half of all admissions for aspiration pneumonia in the 1995 calendar year in the USA and a mortality rate of more than 25% [18]. The United Nations (Department of Economic and Social Affairs – Population Division) notes that by the year 2050 one third of the population in the developed world will be aged over 60 years [19]. In the developing world, this figure will reach 20%. Due to a decline in fertility and an increase in longevity, for the first time in history there will be more elders than young people. The number of individuals affected by oropharyngeal dysphagia looks set to rise.

Although swallowing difficulties increase with advancing age, for many there is the belief that it is an inevitable part of ageing, and thus there is a failure to seek help [12]. Other reasons for not seeking treatment include [13, 20]:

- Poor awareness that treatment for dysphagia was available
- Belief that the dysphagia could not be treated
- Not bothered enough by the problem
- Difficulties with
  - travel to therapy
  - time commitment to therapy or
  - expense of therapy

Impact of Diagnosis of Dysphagia on Prognosis

The prevalence of dysphagia in the hospital setting is not completely known. Data collection processes can yield varying outcomes and likely account for the disparities reported in the literature. For example, dysphagia prevalence was found to be 6.7% in an acute hospital setting, representing patients identified using a nurse-administered dysphagia screening tool, verified by speech pathology and found to require NPO or texture-modified diets. It did not include individuals requiring thickened liquids, however [7]. In contrast, a dysphagia prevalence rate of 0.35% was identified in a large hospital survey database, as described in the United States National Hospital Discharge Survey (NHDS) from 2005 to 2006. In this study, however, the rate of dysphagia was double (0.73% of all hospitalizations) in the age group >75 years old compared to 45–64 years old [6]. Other selected populations are also at much higher risk of having dysphagia, including stroke, and neurodegenerative disease. Also, according to the NHDS study the most common dysphagia-related comorbid conditions were (1) fluid and electrolyte disorder (i.e. dehydration), (2) disease of the esophagus (i.e. reflux or tumor), (3) ischemic stroke, and (4) aspiration pneumonia, accounting for about half of all dysphagia hospitalizations.

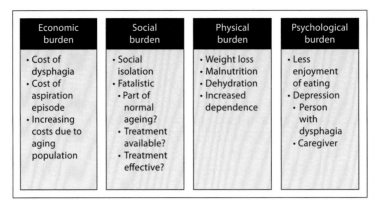

Economic burden	Social burden	Physical burden	Psychological burden
• Cost of dysphagia • Cost of aspiration episode • Increasing costs due to aging population	• Social isolation • Fatalistic • Part of normal ageing? • Treatment available? • Treatment effective?	• Weight loss • Malnutrition • Dehydration • Increased dependence	• Less enjoyment of eating • Depression • Person with dysphagia • Caregiver

Fig. 2. Visual summary: the burden of oropharyngeal dysphagia.

In the hospital setting, dysphagia portends a poor prognosis and ultimately is associated with longer hospital stay, higher costs, and greater risk of mortality. In a study involving the 2003 NHDS, 45% of patients with stroke and dysphagia had hospital length of stay >7 days, compared to 15% of patients with stroke and no dysphagia [21]. Furthermore, only 21% of stroke patients with dysphagia were discharged home compared to 60% of those with no dysphagia. In the more recent study of the NHDS from 2005–2006, the presence of dysphagia in all patients was shown to be associated with 40% increased length of stay (4 days compared to 2.4-day hospitalization in patients without dysphagia) [6]. Mortality was 13 times higher in patients with dysphagia in the rehabilitation setting compared to those with no dysphagia, and 1.8–2.6 times higher during hospitalizations associated with cardiac dysrhythmias and atherosclerosis, respectively.

The consequence of dysphagia in the hospitalized population as described in these studies reflects a number of important conclusions. Namely, (1) dysphagia is underappreciated in the hospital population, and therefore one may surmise that there is some delay in identifying its presence and consequences, (2) these patients are at higher risk of complications such as aspiration pneumonia, malnutrition and potentially death, and (3) certain populations are at higher risk for dysphagia, where there may be a cost-effective role for screening and early intervention.

Burden

Oropharyngeal dysphagia presents many different burdens including physical, social, psychological and economic. These factors are summarized in figure 2. An inability to safely or efficiently eat and drink has pronounced consequences for malnutrition and dehydration. The consequences of dysphagia and malnutrition include: fatigue, aspiration pneumonia, weight loss, dehydration, muscle breakdown, and an overall decline in general health [22]. The threats of sarcopenia and protein-energy malnutrition are ever present for individuals with dysphagia.

In the European study of aged care residents 84% of those surveyed said that eating should be an enjoyable experience; however, only 45% actually considered this to be the case [13]. Individuals reported eating in isolation because they were embarrassed by their swallowing difficulties, and experienced anxiety or panic during mealtimes. Half of those surveyed indicated that swallowing difficulties made life less enjoyable [13].

Dysphagia has been linked with low mood or depression [10]. More than half of the 360 patients in the Ekberg study [13] reported that dysphagia made their life less enjoyable. Feelings of isolation, anxiety and panic at mealtimes, embarrassment and loss of self-esteem significantly reduced quality of life in individuals with dysphagia [13].

With physical changes associated with oropharyngeal dysphagia, there is also an increased physical burden for caregivers. Individuals with dementia often develop dysphagia, and aversive feeding behaviors in this group are common with disease progression. Eating difficulties lead to significant stress for caregivers and health care providers [23, 24]. Caregivers who feel overburdened by behaviors such as turning the head away, pushing the food or feeder away, or accepting food into the mouth but then failing or refusing to swallow, often do not have the physical, emotional or cognitive strategies required to help the person with Alzheimer's disease and dysphagia eat [23]. In fact, the quality of the carer-patient relationship during meals has been noted to account for 32% of variance of food consumed [24]. Where feeding assistance is needed, meals can take as long as 34 min [9]. With increased caregiver burden associated with aversive feeding behavior, there is greater difficulty maintaining the person at home and a higher likelihood of requirement for nursing home placement. It is poignant to note that we can assist people with dysphagia by first assisting their caregivers.

Impact on Hospital Resources

Consequences of oropharyngeal dysphagia can broadly include: weight loss, dehydration, malnutrition, and aspiration pneumonia. The latter is of particular concern due to its link with death. Based on dysphagia present in 0.35% of hospitalized patients, 1.64-day average increased length of stay (considering the 2005–2006 NHDS at 4 days compared to 2.4-day hospitalization in patients without dysphagia), and a conservative estimated USD 2,454 daily fixed and variable costs, the economic impact of dysphagia in the hospital setting was calculated to be USD 547 million annually [6]. This is a low estimate not only

Table 1. Summary of economic costs of oropharyngeal dysphagia [6]

Increased length of stay, days	
Without dysphagia	2.4
With dysphagia	4
Daily fixed and variable costs of dysphagia, USD	2,454
Conservative annual economic cost of dysphagia, USD	547 million

Table 2. Summary of economic costs associated with treatment of aspiration pneumonia, a consequence of oropharyngeal dysphagia

Average length of hospital stay [18], days	16
Mean cost of care per episode of aspiration pneumonia [26], USD	17,000
Cost range for care per episode of aspiration pneumonia depending on number of comorbidities [26], CA	11,000–94,000
Mortality at 1 year [3], %	
With oropharyngeal dysphagia	55
With safe swallowing function	27

because of the lower than expected prevalence, but also because variable costs associated with dysphagia would likely be far greater based on needs for enteral nutrition as well as the consequences of aspiration. Information regarding costs associated with oropharyngeal dysphagia is summarized in table 1.

Treatment of malnutrition, dehydration and aspiration often requires hospital care and medication. Medication costs for i.v. antibiotics have been reported to range from USD 12.70 to 443.70 per course of treatment [25]. In addition to medication, there are also costs associated with staffing and investigative procedures such as X-ray. In a study conducted in the USA in 1995, there were 300,000 admissions for aspiration pneumonia. The mean length of stay was 16.1 days with an average cost of USD 32,000 [18]. In a recent Canadian study, the cost of treatment for aspiration pneumonia increased significantly depending on the number of comorbidities the patient presented with [26]. Although the mean cost per patient was CA ~17,000, it varied from CA 11,000 to 94,000 depending on the number of comorbidities. A team approach to care can minimize costs. For example, the annual costs associated with management of hospitalized chest infections fell from GBP 48.2 million to 26.1 million when speech pathologists were involved in patient care [27]. Information regarding costs associated with aspiration pneumonia is summarized in table 2.

Once oropharyngeal dysphagia is recognized in a hospitalized patient, options generally include rehabilitation, oral diet limitation, as well as recognizing the trade-off between short-term and longer-term enteral nutrition. The use

Cichero · Altman

of the percutaneous endoscopic gastrostomy (PEG) allows for such non-oral feeding, bypassing the oropharyngeal region and supplying required nutrients and hydration directly to the stomach. Therein lies the importance of a team approach to properly diagnose the etiology of dysphagia, and determine prognosis for reasonable recovery.

In the case of stroke patients, the FOOD (Feed Or Ordinary Diet) trials were established to determine the roles of routine oral nutritional supplementation, as well as timing and method of enteral feeding for dysphagia stroke patients [28, 29]. These were multicenter randomized controlled trials involving 4,023 patients at 125 hospitals in 15 countries, whose primary outcome measure was death or Modified Rankin Scale grade 3–5 [28]. In the initial study, only 8% of patients were found to have nutritional deficiency upon admission. In addition to the normal hospital diet, those with additional nutritional supplements did not conclude any meaningful difference in their outcome.

In the sub-study focusing on the potential benefits of enteral feeding, patients were randomized to early enteral feeding versus no tube feeding, and the study found that early tube feeding was associated with an absolute reduction in the risk of death by 5.8% [29]. However, when the study looked at early PEG versus nasogastric feeding, PEG was associated with an absolute increased risk of death in 1%, and an increased risk of death or poor outcome in 7.8%. While it is not immediately apparent, one possibility for this finding is an association with aspiration pneumonia episodes, reported in as many as 10% of patients following or associated with PEG at a cost of USD ~26,000 per admission [18].

However, dysphagia in stroke patients is a unique situation where it resolves in a significant number of patients by day 7 following a stroke. Early intervention with PEG during hospitalization with neurodegenerative disease, postsurgical debilitation and other high-risk groups has not been as thoroughly explored in the literature.

Conclusions

The prevalence of dysphagia is growing with the aging population, and has associations with comorbidities such as stroke and neurodegenerative diseases. In addition to the needs for hydration and nutrition, inability to swallow sufficiently may be associated with significant quality of life impairment and depression. Complications of dysphagia such as aspiration, particularly in the hospitalized population may have catastrophic consequences and add to the burden on healthcare resources.

References

1 Logemann JA: Evaluation and Treatment of Swallowing Disorders, ed 2. Austin, Pro-Ed, 1998, pp 1.

2 Kendall K: Anatomy and physiology of deglutition; in Leonard R, Kendall K (eds): Dysphagia Assessment and Treatment Planning – A Team Approach, ed 2. San Diego, Plural Publishing, 2008, pp 1.

3 Cabre M, Serra-Prat M, Palomera E, et al: Prevalence and prognostic implications of dysphagia in elderly patients with pneumonia. Age Ageing 2010;39:39–45.

4 Stechmiller JK: Early nutritional screening of older adults: a review of nutritional support. J Infus Nurs 2003;26:170–177.

5 Roy N, Stemple J, Merrill RM, et al: Dysphagia in the elderly: preliminary evidence of prevalence, risk factors, and socioemotional effects. Ann Otol Rhinol Laryngol 2007;116:858–865.

6 Altman KW, Yu G-P, Schaeffer SD: Consequence of dysphagia in the hospitalized patient: impact on prognosis and hospital resources. Arch Otolaryngol Head Neck Surg 2010;136:784–789.

7 Cichero JA, Heaton S, Bassett L: Triaging dysphagia: nurse screening for dysphagia in an acute hospital. J Clin Nurs 2009;18:1649–1659.

8 Kayser-Jones K, Pengilly K: Dysphagia among nursing home residents. Geriatr Nurs 1999;20:77–84.

9 Steele CM, Greenwood C, Ens I, et al: Mealtime difficulties in a home for the aged: not just dysphagia. Dysphagia 1997;12:45–50.

10 Holland G, Jayasersekeran V, Pendleton N, et al: Prevalence and symptom profiling of oropharyngeal dysphagia in a community dwelling of an elderly population: self-reporting questionnaire survey. Dis Esophagus 2011; http://onlinelibrary.wiley.com/doi/10.1111/j.1442-2050.2011.01182.x/abstract.

11 Kawashima K, Motohashi Y, Fujishima I: Prevalence of dysphagia among community-dwelling elderly individuals as estimated using a questionnaire for dysphagia screening. Dysphagia 2004;19:266–271.

12 Bloem BR, Lagaay AM, van Beek W, et al: Prevalence of subjective dysphagia in community residents over 87. BMJ 1990;300:721–722.

13 Ekberg O, Hamdy S, Woisard V, et al: Social and psychological burden of dysphagia: Its impact on diagnosis and treatment. Dysphagia 2002;17:139–146.

14 Langdon PC, Lee AH, Binns CW: Dysphagia in acute ischaemic stroke: severity, recovery and relationship to stroke subtype. J Clin Neurosci 2007;14:630–634.

15 Walker RW, Dunn JR, Gray WK: Self-reported dysphagia and its correlates within a prevalent population of people with Parkinson's disease. Dysphagia 2011;26:92–96.

16 Hardiman O: Symptomatic treatment of respiratory and nutritional failure in amyotrophic lateral sclerosis. J Neurol 2000;247:245–251.

17 Barczi SR, Sullivan PA, Robbins J: How should dysphagia care of older adults differ? Establishing optimal practice patterns. Semin Speech Lang 2000;21:347–361.

18 Siddique R, Neslusan CA, Crown WH, et al: A national inpatient cost estimate of percutaneous endoscopic gastrostomy (PEG)-associated aspiration pneumonia. Am J Manag Care 2000;6:490–496.

19 Department of Economic and Social Affairs (Population Division): New York, World Population Ageing: 1950–2050. United Nations Publications, 2001.

20 Turley R, Cohen S: Impact of voice and swallowing problems in the elderly. J Otolaryngol Head Neck Surg 2009;140:33–36.

21 Altman KW, Schaefer SD, Yu GP, et al: The voice and laryngeal dysfunction in stroke: a report from the Neurolaryngology Subcommittee of the American Academy of Otolaryngology-Head and Neck Surgery. Otolaryngol Head Neck Surg 2007;136:873–881.

22 Ney DM, Weiss JM, Kind AJH, et al: Senescent swallowing: impact, strategies and interventions. Nutr Clin Pract 2009;24:395–413.

23 Rivière S, Gillette-Guyonet S, Andrieu S, et al: Cognitive function and caregiver burden: predictive factors for eating behaviours in Alzheimers Disease. Int J Geriatr Psychiatry 2002;17:950–955.

24 Amella EJ: Factors influencing the proportion of food consumed by nursing home residents with dementia. J Am Geriatr Soc 1999;47:879–885.

25 Kadowaki M, Demura Y, Mizuno S, et al: Reappraisal of clindamycin IV monotherapy for treatment of mild-to-moderate aspiration pneumonia in elderly patients. Chest 2005;127:1276–1282.

26 Sutherland JM, Hamm J, Hatcher J: Adjusting casemix payment amounts for inaccurately reported comorbidity data. Health Care Manag Sci 2010;13:65–73.

27 Marsh K, Bertanou E, Suominen H, et al: An economic evaluation of speech and language therapy. Matrix Evidence for the Royal College of Speech and Language Therapists UK, 2010. http://www.rcslt.org/giving_voice/news/matrix_report.

28 The FOOD Trial Collaboration: Routine oral nutritional supplementation for stroke patients in hospital (FOOD): a multi-center randomized controlled trial. Lancet 2005;365:755–763.

29 The FOOD Trial Collaboration: Effect of timing and method of enteral feeding for dysphagic stroke patients (FOOD): a multi-center randomized controlled trial. Lancet 2005;365:764–772.

Cichero J, Clavé P (eds): Stepping Stones to Living Well with Dysphagia.
Nestlé Nutr Inst Workshop Ser, vol 72, pp 13–17,
Nestec Ltd., Vevey/S. Karger AG., Basel, © 2012

The Physiology of Deglutition and the Pathophysiology and Complications of Oropharyngeal Dysphagia

Catriona M. Steele

Toronto Rehabilitation Institute, University of Toronto, and Bloorview Research Institute,
Toronto, ON, Canada

Abstract

The opening session of the 2nd International Conference on Oropharyngeal Dysphagia featured a series of invited talks reviewing the definition of dysphagia, its prevalence and its pathophysiology. The discussion arising from these talks focused heavily on the current underrecognition of dysphagia as a significant concern for older adults, particularly those over 75. The burdens associated with dysphagia in this sector of the population were recognized to be substantial, both in social/psychological terms and in terms of economic consequences for the healthcare system. The importance of developing swallow screening protocols as a routine method for the early identification of dysphagia and aspiration was explored. The idea of launching political initiatives aimed at increasing awareness and the utilization of appropriate dysphagia healthcare codes was also discussed.

The opening session of the 2nd International Conference on Oropharyngeal Dysphagia featured a series of invited talks reviewing the definition of dysphagia, its prevalence and its pathophysiology. Dr. Julie Cichero, from the University of Queensland in Brisbane, Australia, spoke first, defining oropharyngeal dysphagia as difficulty swallowing with two primary functional consequences: poor efficiency leading to inadequate hydration and nutrition, and impaired swallowing safety characterized by aspiration leading to a risk of pneumonia. Dr. Cichero's talk reviewed the prevalence of dysphagia in older adults (those over 60 years of age), citing evidence showing that dysphagia is more likely to be seen in those over the age of 80, particularly those residing in nursing homes, who have reduced functional capacity and are taking multiple medications [1].

She cited data from a number of different studies estimating the prevalence of dysphagia amongst older adults in acute care hospitals to range from 25 to 71%, while comparable figures for nursing homes range from 55 to 68%. Figures for seniors living in the community, derived from surveys were cited to be substantially lower, falling between 11 and 16%. It was noted that underreporting of symptoms may be characteristic of seniors living in the community, who may accept dysphagia as a natural part of growing older.

The issue of dysphagia prevalence was also a main focus of the talk given by Dr. Kenneth Altman from the Mount Sinai School of Medicine in New York. Dr. Altman, an otolaryngologist, described rates of dysphagia amongst adults hospitalized at his institution, ranging from 12% in those under 45 to 73% in those over the age of 75 [2, 3]. Dr. Altman argued that dysphagia is an underrecognized condition that contributes to a 40% increased length of stay and 13-fold increased mortality during hospitalization for elderly patients.

These two talks elicited questions and comments from the audience regarding the fact that dysphagia appears to be underrecognized or underdocumented in the geriatric population. One possible reason for this is failure on the part of physicians to implement the appropriate medical codes to capture and note dysphagia as part of a patient's condition. Dr. Pere Clavé pointed out that the World Health Organization has recently established a specific code for oropharyngeal dysphagia within its International Classification of Diseases (ICD-10) system (http://www.who.int/classifications/icd/en). He acknowledged that dysphagia has not traditionally been considered a disease, but rather a symptom or component of many other disease and injury conditions, but argued that our understanding and appreciation of dysphagia prevalence and epidemiology would be significantly advanced if initiatives were taken to encourage physicians to use the oropharyngeal dysphagia code in their medical reports. Dr. Clavé mentioned that the European Society for Swallowing Disorders would be launching an initiative along these lines called 'Dysphagia Day'. Another audience member, Ms. Carola Granholm, a dietitian from Stockholm, pointed out that similar concerns have been raised regarding the recognition and awareness of malnutrition in the elderly, and that ESPEN, the European Society for Parenteral and Enteral Nutrition has been working for several years to improve awareness about malnutrition in the EU. She argued that awareness may need to be raised to the political level if the necessary financial resources are going to be made available to properly address the burden of dysphagia for our aging population.

The question of the burden of dysphagia was also addressed in Dr. Cichero's talk. She argued eloquently that dysphagia results in social, psychological and financial burden. With respect to social concerns, dysphagia frequently leads to patients eating in isolation. Dr. Altman concurred, arguing that this robs patients of the very basic function of 'breaking bread together' that is so integral to our lives. Dr. Cichero cited studies showing a strong correlation between dysphagia and depression, and reports that up to half of nursing home residents report that eating is no longer enjoyable and that requiring assistance to eat is a burden. She further pointed out that many patients find texture-modified foods and thickened liquids to be unpalatable, and that recommendations for enteral feeding and nil-by-mouth status lead to even greater feelings of social isolation.

These considerations prompted comments from the audience regarding the need for follow-up assessment for adults who have been discharged from acute care back into community or nursing-home settings on texture-modified diets. A previous study by Groher and McKaig [4] was cited as evidence that many individuals in nursing homes may be able to tolerate upgrades from texture-modified diets that were recommended during their acute care stays. Dr. Altman further argued for the consideration of allowing some safe oral intake, as tolerated, in older adults who may need enteral feeding to achieve optimal nutrition. He mentioned that many of the individuals he sees who are unable to meet their nutritional needs orally are still able to manage some safe swallowing; from a quality of life perspective, he argued that allowing some oral intake on compassionate grounds could restore some normalcy to these patients' lives with respect to the important social benefits of eating with their family and friends.

With respect to the economic burden of dysphagia, the available statistics cited by both Drs. Cichero and Altman dealt primarily with the costs of treating aspiration pneumonia as a sequel of dysphagia. A recent Canadian study [5] cited costs per case of USD 17,240 to treat aspiration pneumonia, with British estimates of annual costs reaching as high as GBP 48 million under standard care conditions. Importantly, the British figures showed cost reductions in the order of GBP 22 million when speech pathology care for dysphagia is provided.

These considerations of dysphagia burden led to questions from the audience about the optimum method of intervening to reduce the negative impact of dysphagia. Dr. Michael Jedwab from Nestlé Healthcare Nutrition proposed that early identification and diagnosis would serve to stop the negative cycle of malnutrition and pneumonia risk that seems to spiral out of control when dysphagia is not recognized. He asked whether this cascade should perhaps not be attributed so much to lack of recognition but rather to a lack of simple and efficient screening tools that could be used to identify individuals at risk upon entry to hospital or at physicians' offices in the community.

Dr. Cichero agreed that screening can play a very important part in raising the awareness and improving the recognition of dysphagia. She reported that an increase in the number of patients identified as having dysphagia had resulted from the implementation of a nurse screening tool at the Royal Brisbane Hospital [6]. Dr. Rosemary Martino from the University of Toronto concurred, citing work by Hinchey and colleagues showing that the implementation of dysphagia screening protocols leads to a 3-fold reduction in the rate of hospital-acquired pneumonia [7]. She pointed out, however, that implementing screening programs is not always easy and a number of barriers may be encountered. Dr. Martino reported that her work on swallow screening protocols implemented by nursing shows that uptake takes time, and that creating a culture in which nurses accept the role of swallow screening, incorporate the necessary skills into their practice and develop comfort with having this new task as part of their repertoire may require as long as a year. She argued for the importance of mentoring and providing support to nursing staff to implement these kinds of changes.

With respect to barriers to implementing screening programs, Dr. Altman pointed out that investing resources in early identification and screening programs for any disease condition is recognized to be a good investment, but that unfortunately health system budgets frequently fail to invest in such long-term planning, based on pressures that direct money toward more immediate concerns. Financial barriers were also mentioned as a concern with respect to implementing programs to monitor patients upon discharge from acute care back to community settings.

The remaining talks in the opening session of the conference addressed the specifics of the pathophysiology of dysphagia and aspiration. Dr. Shaheen Hamdy from Manchester, UK, reviewed the neurophysiology of swallowing, and described methods for mapping the swallowing neural pathways, both sensory and motor, that are used in his laboratory. Dr. Clave, from Mataro in Spain, described issues related to the timing of the swallow response and the reconfiguration of the oropharynx from a respiratory passage to an alimentary passage. Dr. Cichero, along with Dr. Eric Verin from Rouen, France, discussed issues of respiratory-swallow coordination.

The discussion concluded with a brief exploration of the extent to which clinicians might access dysphagia assessment methods that more fully reveal abnormalities in swallowing neurophysiology. Dr. Hamdy acknowledged that there are very limited options in terms of clinical tools for evaluating the integrity of sensory pathways in swallowing, and reported that advanced methods such as tractography are unlikely to become available on a large scale basis due to cost. He argued that these sophisticated methods would be best used to study small clusters of patients to understand the central mechanisms involved in their dysphagia, and then to extrapolate the findings to other patient groups.

References

1 Cabre M, Serra-Prat M, Palomera E, et al: Prevalence and prognostic implications of dysphagia in elderly patients with pneumonia. Age Ageing 2010;39:39–45.
2 Altman KW, Yu GP, Schaefer SD: Consequence of dysphagia in the hospitalized patient: impact on prognosis and hospital resources. Arch Otolaryngol Head Neck Surg 2010;136:784–789.
3 Altman KW: Dysphagia evaluation and care in the hospital setting: the need for protocolization. Otolaryngol Head Neck Surg 2011;145:895–898.
4 Groher ME, McKaig TN: Dysphagia and dietary levels in skilled nursing facilities. J Am Geriatr Soc 1995;43:528–532.

5   Sutherland JM, Hamm J, Hatcher J:
    Adjusting case mix payment amounts for
    inaccurately reported comorbidity data.
    Health Care Manag Sci 2010;13:65–73.
6   Cichero JA, Heaton S, Bassett L: Triaging
    dysphagia: nurse screening for dysphagia in
    an acute hospital. J Clin Nurs 2009;18:1649–
    1659.

7   Hinchey JA, Shephard T, Furie K, et al:
    Formal dysphagia screening protocols pre-
    vent pneumonia. Stroke 2005;36:1972–1976.

Cichero J, Clavé P (eds): Stepping Stones to Living Well with Dysphagia.
Nestlé Nutr Inst Workshop Ser, vol 72, pp 19–31,
Nestec Ltd., Vevey/S. Karger AG., Basel, © 2012

Identifying Vulnerable Patients: Role of the EAT-10 and the Multidisciplinary Team for Early Intervention and Comprehensive Dysphagia Care

Kala Kaspar[a] · Olle Ekberg[b]

[a]Global Medical Affairs, Nestlé HealthCare Nutrition, Nestlé Health Science SA, Vevey, Switzerland;
[b]Department of Diagnostic Radiology, Skåne Hospital, Lund University, Malmö, Sweden

Abstract

There is underdiagnosis and low awareness of dysphagia despite that the condition is modifiable and poorly managed symptoms diminish psychological well-being and overall quality of life. Frontline clinicians are in a unique position to be alert to the high prevalence of swallowing difficulty among elderly, evaluate and identify those who need intervention, and assure that individuals receive appropriate care. Proper diagnosis and treatment of oral-pharyngeal dysphagia involves a multidisciplinary healthcare team effort and starts with systematic screening of at-risk patients. The presence of a medical condition such as acute stroke, head and neck cancer, head trauma, Alzheimer's disease, Parkinson's disease, pneumonia or bronchitis is adequate basis for predicting high risk. Systematic screening of dysphagia and resulting malnutrition among at-risk older adults is justified in an effort to avoid pneumonia and is recommended by clinical practice guidelines. Systematic screening with a validated method (e.g. the 10-item Eating Assessment Tool, EAT-10) as part of a comprehensive care protocol enables multidisciplinary teams to more effectively manage the condition, reduce the economic and societal burden, and improve patient quality of life. In fact, care settings with a systematic dysphagia screening program attain significantly better patient outcomes including reduced cases of pneumonia (by 55%) and reduced hospital length of stay.   Copyright © 2012 Nestec Ltd., Vevey/S. Karger AG, Basel

Introduction

Frontline clinicians are in a unique position to be alert to the high prevalence of swallowing difficulty among elderly, evaluate and identify those who need intervention, and assure that individuals are appropriately treated [1]. While the condition is modifiable, too often there is a lack of diagnosis and early management of dysphagia [2]. Proper diagnosis and treatment of oral-pharyngeal dysphagia involves a multidisciplinary healthcare team effort and starts with systematic screening of at-risk patients.

Individuals with Dysphagia Suffer Symptoms That Diminish Quality of Life

Dysphagia is a symptom, the perception that there is an impediment to the normal passage of swallowed material [4].

Results of a landmark pan-European survey from 1999 characterize the impact dysphagia has on eating pattern, psychological well-being and overall quality of life in older adults. Individuals included in the survey were selected based on known symptoms of dysphagia. A total of 360 people cared for in nursing homes and hospitals in Germany, France, Spain and the UK were interviewed using a 28-item questionnaire [2]. Qualitative interviews with a total of 28 healthcare professionals were conducted in parallel. Sixty-seven percent of respondents had underlying medical conditions as a source of dysphagia, including stroke, Parkinson's disease, Alzheimer's disease, multiple sclerosis and head and neck injuries [2]. More than half of the individuals were between 60 and 79 years of age, i.e. the age range during which a good quality of life can still be expected [2].

In the people interviewed, a few specific symptoms were common, related to eating/drinking being painful, stressful, burdensome, and no longer pleasurable. Namely, 55% experienced 'food sticking in the throat or choking on food', and almost as many (46%) suffered from 'persistent cough or sore throat' related to an inability to swallow liquids [2]. The 'inability to swallow liquids' and 'loss of appetite' were reported by nearly 40%.

Over 50% of the individuals with known symptoms of dysphagia indicated that they ate less due to their dysphagia symptoms, while 44% reported weight loss over the previous 12 months [2]. One third of patients reported being hungry and thirsty even after their meal [2]. Dysphagia is now known to be one of the identifiable and treatable causes of malnutrition and/or dehydration. Accordingly, clinical practice guidelines of premier associations recommend early identification of dysphagia as well as malnutrition and dehydration risk, and appropriate interventions [5–11].

While eating and drinking are normally social and pleasurable experiences, 55% of respondents reported that swallowing problems 'made life less enjoyable' [2]. The added 'embarrassment' and 'anxiety or panic during mealtimes', experienced by 37 and 41%, respectively, of patients because of swallowing difficulties, can lead patients to 'avoid eating with others', which was reported by 36% of respondents [2]. All of these psychological factors may lead to reduced fluid and nutritional intakes, and increased risk of malnutrition and dehydration. Clearly, individuals with unmanaged dysphagia suffer a loss of the pleasure of eating.

Collectively, this study suggests a correlation between dysphagia and reduced social and psychological health. Hence, reduced quality of life is a potential consequence of poorly managed dysphagia.

Systematic Screening of At-Risk Patients Is Justified for the Early Management of Dysphagia

The pan-European study results also reveal underdiagnosis and low awareness of dysphagia, despite the high prevalence and negative impact of swallowing problems. Only 40% of the individuals with dysphagia in formal care settings included in this survey acknowledged receiving a confirmed diagnosis of dysphagia [2]. Two thirds received no treatment despite there being options available, such as changing food consistency, specifically designed nutritional products, adaptation of eating position and swallowing exercises [2]. If not asked by health care professionals about swallowing difficulties, less than half would mention their symptoms [2].

More recent evidence suggests a lack of formal dysphagia screening protocols being used, even among poststroke patients, in which advantages of systematic screening and early intervention with modified liquids and foods have been repeatedly demonstrated (as summarized in table 1). A prospective study of 15 US acute care hospitals found that only 40% of the care settings have a systematic screening program in place [12]. Among the broader at-risk population, researchers estimate that only 25% of individuals in an institutional care setting who have dysphagia are diagnosed with the disorder [13].

In care settings with a systematic dysphagia screening program, significantly better patient outcomes were observed including: reduced cases of pneumonia (by 55%) and reduced hospital length of stay [12]. Associated with these outcomes is the potential to reduce costs and the risk of early mortality common among those who develop pneumonia [12]. Based on the substantial benefits possible, clinical practice guidelines of premier associations recommend dysphagia screening among at-risk patients (as summarized in table 2). For example, the American College of Chest Physicians (ACCP) clinical practice guidelines recommend oral-pharyngeal swallowing evaluation for:

- 'Patients who are at high risk for aspiration (that might be silent) having conditions including: Cerebrovascular disease (stroke), Head & neck cancer; Head trauma; Parkinson's disease, Alzheimer's disease' (grade of recommendation B) [5].
- 'Patients with cough that is related to pneumonia and bronchitis' (grade of recommendation B) [5].

Table 1. Clinical study evidence summary: improved patient outcomes achieved with systematic screening and early intervention for dysphagia

Study population	Age	Intervention
Poststroke patients	Intervention: 69.8 ± 12.5 years Control: 71.4 ± 12.7 years	Individuals were systematically screened and received intervention under the direction of the speech language pathologist including: • Swallowing interventions were based on the findings of the clinical examination and VFSS, administered at baseline and at follow-up if necessary • Direct swallowing exercises Examples: effortful swallowing and supraglottic swallow technique Duration: every working day for a month or daily for the duration of the hospital stay (if less than a month) • Appropriate dietary modification
Poststroke patients	75.2 ± 1.5 years	Individuals were systematically screened and received intervention with modified liquids and foods as appropriate
Poststroke patients	NA	Individuals were systematically screened and received intervention from a multidisciplinary team including: • Swallowing interventions were based on the findings of the clinical examination and endoscopy • Individualized therapy program • Appropriate dietary modification
Patients with neurogenic conditions	Intervention: 49.3 years (range = 22–86 years) Control: 46.1 years (range = 22–77 years)	Individuals were systematically screened and received intervention from a multidisciplinary team including: • Swallowing interventions were based on the findings of the clinical examination and VFSS • Swallow therapy included oromotor exercises, thermal stimulation, etc. Example: supraglottic swallow technique • Appropriate dietary modification

VFSS = Videofluoroscopic swallow study; NA = not available.

Control	Duration and follow-up	Outcomes	p value	Reference
Individuals received conventional care under the direction of the attending physician including: • Physicians referred patients to the speech pathology service if deemed appropriate • Treatment, if offered, consisted mainly of precautions for safe swallowing during daily meals and snacks: 1. Feeding supervision 2. Positioning during feeding 3. Slowed rate of feeding • Swallowing function is assessed by VFSS if prescribed by the attending physician (applied to 27% of patients)	6-month follow-up	Systematic screening and early intervention with a comprehensive program of direct swallowing exercises and appropriate dietary modification:		26
		Increased proportion of stroke patients who recovered swallowing	0.02	
		Increased proportion of stroke patients who returned to a normal diet	0.04	
		Decreased proportion of patients who had a clinical complication (46 vs. 63% for usual care, relative risk 0.73)	0.05	
		Decreased proportion of patients who developed pneumonia (26 vs. 47% for usual care, relative risk 0.56)	0.003	
No systematic screening and early intervention program in place	duration of hospital-ization	Incidence of aspiration pneumonia among post-stroke patients was reduced from 6.7% to 0% in year 2 (100% relative risk reduction)	NA	27 28
		Potential to realize marginal cost savings	NA	29
No systematic screening and early intervention program in place	90-day follow-up	Reduce mortality (7.4 vs. 4.2%)	NA	30
		Reduce incidence of pneumonia (9.0 vs. 2.8%)	<0.05	
		Cost savings on antibiotics (50% savings)	NA	
No systematic screening and early intervention program in place	Intervention: 31.9 days (range = 3–130 days) Control: 41.1 days (range = 4– 45 days)	Improve nutrient intakes (miss daily caloric goals by only 97 vs. 488.5 kcal)	0.05	3
		Avoid weight loss (mean weight gain of 1.41 kg vs. mean weight loss of 2.8 kg)	0.02	

Table 2. List of clinical practice guidelines from premier associations that recommend dysphagia screening among at-risk patients

Title	Body
Cough and aspiration of food and liquids due to oral-pharyngeal dysphagia: ACCP evidence-based clinical practice guidelines	ACCP [5]
Disease-Specific Care Certification Program: Stroke Performance Measurement Implementation Guide	Joint Commission [15]
Multiple sclerosis. National clinical guideline for diagnosis and management in primary and secondary care	National Institute for Health and Clinical Excellence [16]
World Gastroenterology Organization Practice Guidelines: Dysphagia	World Gastroenterology Organization [4]
Parkinson's disease in the long-term care setting	American Medical Directors Association [17]
Dementia care practice recommendations for assisted living residences and nursing homes	Alzheimer's Association [6]
Diagnosis and management of head and neck cancer. A national clinical guideline	Scottish Intercollegiate Guidelines Network [18]
Traumatic brain injury: diagnosis, acute management and rehabilitation	New Zealand Guidelines Group [19]
Management of patients with stroke: identification and management of dysphagia. A national clinical guideline	Scottish Intercollegiate Guidelines Network [20]
National clinical guidelines for stroke: the Intercollegiate Stroke Working Party	Royal College of Physicians [9]
Nutritional management in long-term care: development of a clinical guideline	Council for Nutritional Strategies in Long-Term Care [21]

The ACCP also recommends, 'Further evaluation, including a chest radiograph and a nutritional assessment, should be considered in patients with cough or conditions associated with aspiration' (grade of recommendation B) [5].

Screening serves to facilitate targeted referral of persons at dysphagia risk to dysphagia specialists for further assessment and to initiate appropriate interventions. In principle, a good screening tool will be quick, easy, and validated [14].

Results of the pan-European survey and other studies point to the need for active detection and heightened awareness of dysphagia among at-risk patient populations. The 10-item Eating Assessment Tool (EAT-10; as shown in fig. 1)

EAT-10:
A Swallowing Screening Tool

Nestlé Nutrition Institute

LAST NAME	FIRST NAME	SEX	AGE	DATE

OBJECTIVE:

EAT-10 helps to measure swallowing difficulties.
It may be important for you to talk with your physician about treatment options for symptoms.

A. INSTRUCTIONS:

Answer each question by writing the number of points in the boxes.
To what extent do you experience the following problems?

1 My swallowing problem has caused me to lose weight.

0 = no problem
1
2
3
4 = severe problem

2 My swallowing problem interferes with my ability to go out for meals.

0 = no problem
1
2
3
4 = severe problem

3 Swallowing liquids takes extra effort.

0 = no problem
1
2
3
4 = severe problem

4 Swallowing solids takes extra effort.

0 = no problem
1
2
3
4 = severe problem

5 Swallowing pills takes extra effort.

0 = no problem
1
2
3
4 = severe problem

6 Swallowing is painful.

0 = no problem
1
2
3
4 = severe problem

7 The pleasure of eating is affected by my swallowing.

0 = no problem
1
2
3
4 = severe problem

8 When I swallow food sticks in my throat.

0 = no problem
1
2
3
4 = severe problem

9 I cough when I eat.

0 = no problem
1
2
3
4 = severe problem

10 Swallowing is stressful.

0 = no problem
1
2
3
4 = severe problem

B. SCORING:

Add up the number of points and write your total score in the boxes.
Total Score (max. 40 points)

C. WHAT TO DO NEXT:

If the EAT-10 score is 3 or higher, you may have problems swallowing efficiently and safely. We recommend discussing the EAT-10 results with a physician.

Reference: The validity and reliability of EAT-10 has been determined.
Belafsky PC, Mouadeb DA, Rees CJ, Pryor JC, Postma GN, Allen J, Leonard RJ. Validity and Reliability of the Eating Assessment Tool (EAT-10). Annals of Otology Rhinology & Laryngology 2008;117(12):919-924.

www.nestlenutrition-institute.org

Fig. 1. The EAT-10, a validated dysphagia screening tool.

Identifying Vulnerable Patients

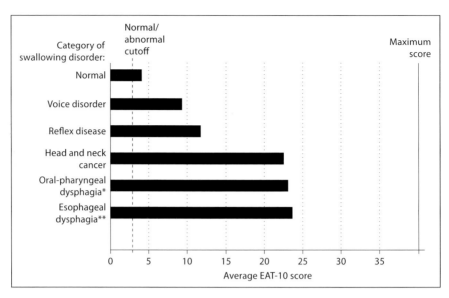

Fig. 2. Typical EAT-10 scores by type of swallow impairment. * Mostly patients with a diagnosis of stroke or progressive neurologic disease (Parkinson's disease, etc.). ** Mostly patients with a diagnosis of esophageal motility disorders, neoplasia, webs, strictures or rings.

is a screening tool specifically designed to address the clinical need for a rapidly administered and easily scored questionnaire to assess dysphagia symptom severity. The tool is applicable to a broad range of dysphagic patients, those with oral-pharyngeal dysphagia as well as those with esophageal dysphagia. It was developed by a multidisciplinary group of dysphagia experts who contributed a set of questions based on existing evidence, clinical experience and established questionnaires. An initial list of 35 questions was shortened to 20 by voting and further amended to 10 items selected based on strong test-retest correlations. The EAT-10 is rapidly self-administered and can be completed in <2 min [22]. An EAT-10 score >3 is abnormal and indicates the presence of swallowing difficulties. For the subgroup with oral-pharyngeal dysphagia, who were primarily patients with a diagnosis of stroke or progressive neurologic disease (Parkinson's disease, etc.), the average EAT-10 score was 23.1 ± 12.2. Other average EAT-10 scores typical of specific categories of swallowing disorders are shown in figure 2.

In a study among dysphagia patients receiving care in an outpatient clinic (mean age of 65 ± 16 years), the EAT-10 displayed excellent internal consistency, test-retest reproducibility, and criterion-based validity [22]. Further research among patients from acute care, long-term care, and primary care settings demonstrated that the EAT-10 is useful as a clinician- and self-administered test, easy to understand for the majority (95.4%) of patients, quick to perform having a mean completion time of <4 min, and able to differentiate patients at risk for dysphagia from those with a normal swallow [23]. The EAT-10 form can be accessed at http://www.nestlenutrition-institute.org/ PracticalTools/Documents/test1.pdf.

Investigators report that a large percentage of elderly in formal care settings who suffer from swallowing problems do not receive proper diagnosis (60%) and timely treatment (66%) [2]. This is exposing a vulnerable group of the population to the possibility of dehydration and/or malnutrition, with the long-term social, psychological and medical consequences that can affect quality of life.

A systematic approach to early diagnosis can help prevent long-term consequences and improve quality of life for those suffering from dysphagia. Together, early screening and targeted in-depth assessments allow the multidisciplinary team to plan and initiate interventions as well as establish the baseline for follow-up. Implementation of a comprehensive dysphagia management protocol (such as shown in figure 3) promotes formal screening with validated methods and appropriate early management in at-risk individuals, important for optimizing clinical as well as economic outcomes.

Proper Management of Dysphagia Patients Requires a Multidisciplinary Team Effort

In a stepwise, integrated manner, the multidisciplinary team acts to identify dysphagia risk, conduct clinical assessment and instrumental diagnostic tests for dysphagia, intervene with therapeutic strategies and provide follow-up care.

Step 1: Evaluate for Swallowing Difficulty: Identify Dysphagia Problems Early in Vulnerable Patients
The first step in the process of dysphagia patient care is recognizing the vulnerable patient. The patient's clinical history, physical examination, and results of a basic screening test are useful at this stage [4]. The patient's clinical history and specifically the presence of a certain medical condition (e.g. acute stroke, head and neck cancer, head trauma, Alzheimer's disease, Parkinson's disease) is adequate basis for predicting high risk and the need for evaluation [5]. As noted in the ACCP clinical practice guidelines, it is also important to screen patients with pneumonia or bronchitis for dysphagia risk [5]. Be aware that older adults are more vulnerable to dysphagia, as the swallowing mechanism is altered among otherwise healthy older adults, what is termed 'presbyphagia'. With additional stressors such as acute illness and use of certain medications, an older individual can begin to experience dysphagia [24].

Step 2: Evaluate for Oral-Pharyngeal Dysphagia: Identify Aspiration Risk and Appropriate Diet Prescription
Based on the evidence obtained by clinical history, physical examination, and a basic screening test (e.g. EAT-10), oral-pharyngeal dysphagia may be suspected,

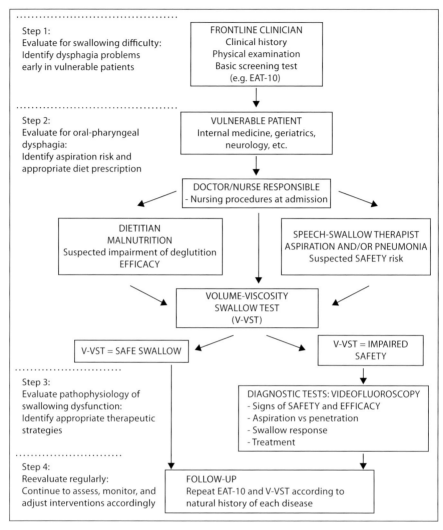

Step 1:
Evaluate for swallowing difficulty:
Identify dysphagia problems
early in vulnerable patients

FRONTLINE CLINICIAN
Clinical history
Physical examination
Basic screening test
(e.g. EAT-10)

Step 2:
Evaluate for oral-pharyngeal
dysphagia:
Identify aspiration risk and
appropriate diet prescription

VULNERABLE PATIENT
Internal medicine, geriatrics,
neurology, etc.

DOCTOR/NURSE RESPONSIBLE
- Nursing procedures at admission

DIETITIAN
MALNUTRITION
Suspected impairment of deglutition
EFFICACY

SPEECH-SWALLOW THERAPIST
ASPIRATION AND/OR PNEUMONIA
Suspected SAFETY risk

VOLUME-VISCOSITY
SWALLOW TEST
(V-VST)

V-VST = SAFE SWALLOW

V-VST = IMPAIRED
SAFETY

Step 3:
Evaluate pathophysiology of
swallowing dysfunction:
Identify appropriate therapeutic
strategies

DIAGNOSTIC TESTS: VIDEOFLUOROSCOPY
- Signs of SAFETY and EFFICACY
- Aspiration vs penetration
- Swallow response
- Treatment

Step 4:
Reevaluate regularly:
Continue to assess, monitor, and
adjust interventions accordingly

FOLLOW-UP
Repeat EAT-10 and V-VST according to
natural history of each disease

Fig. 3. Comprehensive dysphagia patient management protocol. Adapted from Clavé et al. [25].

and subsequently the physician will order evaluation by the multidisciplinary healthcare team. The dietitian may conduct a comprehensive nutrition assessment, determining the nutritional risk and needs of the individual. The nurse will provide direct patient care and may conduct relevant procedures (e.g. record daily fluid intake). The dysphagia specialist (specially trained speech-language pathologist, logopedist, etc.) will determine aspiration risk and identify the appropriate diet prescription (the texture of solids, and the volume and viscosity of liquids). The volume-viscosity swallow test (V-VST) is a sensitive clinical method to identify patients with oral-pharyngeal dysphagia whose swallowing could be improved by intervention with liquids of specific volume and viscosity [25]. An important feature of the V-VST is that it can help improve the detection of swallowing dysfunction, including silent aspiration. Widespread use of this evidence-based method will facilitate appropriate early management oral-pharyngeal dysphagia.

Step 3: Evaluate Pathophysiology of Swallowing Dysfunction: Identify Appropriate Therapeutic Strategies
Based on the clinical evaluation of oral-pharyngeal dysphagia and aspiration (e.g. positive V-VST results), diagnostic tests may be ordered. Videofluoroscopic swallowing study is the gold standard method for identifying the pathophysiology of the dysfunction and appropriate therapeutic strategies (e.g. direct swallowing exercises). Members of the multidisciplinary team work together to assure the comprehensive needs of the patient are met.

Step 4: Reevaluate Regularly: Continue to Assess, Monitor, and Adjust Interventions Accordingly
Regularly assess dysphagia severity, monitoring the effects of treatment and adjusting interventions accordingly. Regular use of the EAT-10 (e.g. on each patient visit) is a practical way to assess changes in symptom severity and guide patient care.

Conclusions

The symptoms of dysphagia and resulting malnutrition are treatable life-threatening conditions that validated screening methods can help to quickly and easily identify. Earlier nutrition intervention coupled with systematic screening enables multidisciplinary teams to more effectively manage these under-diagnosed conditions, reduce the economic and societal burden, and improve patient quality of life.

References

1   Cichero JA, Heaton S, Bassett L: Triaging dysphagia: nurse screening for dysphagia in an acute hospital. J Clin Nurs 2009;18:1649–1659.
2   Ekberg O, Hamdy S, Woisard V, et al: Social and psychological burden of dysphagia: its impact on diagnosis and treatment. Dysphagia 2002;17:139–146.
3   Martens L, Cameron T, Simonsen M: Effects of a multidisciplinary management program on neurologically impaired patients with dysphagia. Dysphagia 1990;5:147–151.
4   World Gastroenterology Organization Practice Guidelines: Dysphagia 2007. http://www.worldgastroenterology.org/assets/downloads/en/pdf/guidelines/08_dysphagia.pdf.

5 American College of Chest Physicians (ACCP), Smith Hammond CA, Goldstein LB: Cough and aspiration of food and liquids due to oral-pharyngeal dysphagia: ACCP evidence-based clinical practice guidelines. Chest 2006;129(suppl 1):154S–168S.

6 Alzheimer's Association, Tilly J, Reed P: Dementia Care Practice Recommendations for Assisted Living Residences and Nursing Homes. Washington, Alzheimer's Association, 2006.

7 National Institute for Health and Clinical Excellence (NICE), National Collaborating Center for Acute Care: Nutrition Support in Adults: Oral Nutrition Support, Enteral Tube Feeding and Parenteral Nutrition. London, National Collaborating Center for Acute Care, 2005.

8 Registered Nurses Association of Ontario (RNAO) & Heart and Stroke Foundation of Ontario (HSFO): Stroke Assessment: Across the Continuum of Care. Toronto, Registered Nurses Association of Ontario, 2005.

9 Royal College of Physicians: National Clinical Guidelines for Stroke, ed 2. London, The Intercollegiate Stroke Working Party, 2004.

10 Rotilio G, Berni Canani R, Branca F, et al: Nutritional recommendations for the management of stroke patients. Riv Ital Nutr Parenter Enter 2004;22:227–236.

11 Miller RG, Rosenberg JA, Gelinas DF, et al: Practice parameter: the care of the patient with amyotrophic lateral sclerosis (an evidence-based review): report of the Quality Standards Subcommittee of the American Academy of Neurology: ALS Practice Parameters Task Force. Neurology 1999;52:1311–1323.

12 Hinchey JA, Shephard T, Furie K, et al, Stroke Practice Improvement Network Investigators: Formal dysphagia screening protocols prevent pneumonia. Stroke 2005;36:1972–1976.

13 Kayser-Jones J, Pengilly K: Dysphagia among nursing home residents. Geriatr Nurs 1999;20:77–82.

14 Jones JM: The methodology of nutritional screening and assessment tools. J Hum Nutr Diet 2002;15:59–71.

15 Joint Commission: Disease-Specific Care Certification Program: Stroke Performance Measurement Implementation Guide, ed 2, version 2.A; updated October 2008.

16 National Institute for Health and Clinical Excellence (NICE), National Collaborating Center for Chronic Conditions: Multiple Sclerosis. National Clinical Guideline for Diagnosis and Management in Primary and Secondary Care. London, National Institute for Health and Clinical Excellence, 2004.

17 American Medical Directors Association (AMDA): Parkinson's Disease in the Long-Term Care Setting. Columbia, American Medical Directors Association, 2002.

18 Scottish Intercollegiate Guidelines Network (SIGN). Diagnosis and Management of Head and Neck Cancer. A National Clinical Guideline. Edinburgh, Scottish Intercollegiate Guidelines Network, 2006.

19 New Zealand Guidelines Group (NZGG): Traumatic Brain Injury: Diagnosis, Acute Management and Rehabilitation. Wellington, New Zealand Guidelines Group, 2006.

20 Scottish Intercollegiate Guidelines Network (SIGN): Management of Patients with Stroke: Identification and Management of Dysphagia. A National Clinical Guideline. Edinburgh, Scottish Intercollegiate Guidelines Network, 2004.

21 Council for Nutritional Strategies in Long-Term Care, Thomas DR, Ashmen W, Morley JE, Evans WJ: Nutritional management in long-term care: development of a clinical guideline. J Gerontol A Biol Sci Med Sci 2000;55:M725–M734.

22 Belafsky PC, Mouadeb DA, Rees CJ, et al: Validity and reliability of the Eating Assessment Tool (EAT-10). Ann Otol Rhinol Laryngol 2008;117:919–924.

23 Burgos R, Sarto B, Segurola H, et al: Translation and validation of the Spanish version of the Eating Assessment Tool-10 (EAT-10) for the screening of dysphagia; in 33 Eur Soc Clin Nutr Metab Congr, Gothenburg, September 2011.

24 Ney DM, Weiss JM, Kind AJ, Robbins J: Senescent swallowing: impact, strategies, and interventions. Nutr Clin Pract 2009;24:395–413.

25 Clave P, Arreola V, Romea M, Medina L, et al: Accuracy of the volume-viscosity swallow test for clinical screening of oropharyngeal dysphagia and aspiration. Clin Nutr 2008;27:806–815.

26 Carnaby G, Hankey GJ, Pizzi J: Behavioural intervention for dysphagia in acute stroke: a randomised controlled trial. Lancet Neurol 2006;5:31–37.

27 Odderson IR, Keaton JC, McKenna BS: Swallow management in patients on an acute stroke pathway: quality is cost effective. Arch Phys Med Rehabil 1995;76:1130–1133.

28 Doggett DL, Tappe KA, Mitchell MD: Prevention of pneumonia in elderly stroke patients by systematic diagnosis and treatment of dysphagia: an evidence-based comprehensive analysis of the literature. Dysphagia 2001;16:279–295.

29 Agency for Healthcare Research and Quality (AHRQ): Diagnosis and treatment of swallowing disorders (dysphagia) in acute care stroke patients. 1999. http://www.ahrq. gov/clinic/tp/dysphtp.htm; Supplemental analysis: cost-effectiveness analysis of a dysphagia diagnosis and treatment program. 1999. http://www.ncbi.nlm.nih.gov/books/ bv.fcgi?rid=hstat1.section.12017.

30 Ickenstein GW, Riecker A, Höhlig C, et al: Pneumonia and in-hospital mortality in the context of neurogenic oropharyngeal dysphagia (NOD) in stroke and a new NOD step-wise concept. J Neurol 2010;257:1492–1499.

Detection

Cichero J, Clavé P (eds): Stepping Stones to Living Well with Dysphagia.
Nestlé Nutr Inst Workshop Ser, vol 72, pp 33–42,
Nestec Ltd., Vevey/S. Karger AG., Basel, © 2012

The Volume-Viscosity Swallow Test for Clinical Screening of Dysphagia and Aspiration

Laia Rofes[a] · Viridiana Arreola[b] · Pere Clavé[a,b]

[a]Centro de Investigación Biomédica en Red de Enfermedades Hepáticas y Digestivas (CIBERehd),
Instituto de Salud Carlos III, [b]Unitat d'Exploracions Funcionals Digestives, Hospital de Mataró,
Barcelona, Spain

Abstract

Background: Oropharyngeal dysphagia (OD) is a major complaint among many patients with neurological diseases and in the elderly, but is often underdiagnosed. The volume-viscosity swallow test (V-VST) is a bedside method to screen patients for dysphagia. **Methods:** The V-VST was designed to identify clinical signs of impaired efficacy (labial seal, oral and pharyngeal residue, and piecemeal deglutition) and impaired safety of swallow (voice changes, cough and decrease in oxygen saturation ≥3%). It starts with nectar viscosity and increasing bolus volume, then liquid and finally pudding viscosity in a progression of increasing difficulty to protect patients from aspiration. **Results:** The V-VST allows quick, safe and accurate screening for OD in hospitalized and independently living patients with multiple etiologies. The V-VST presents a sensitivity of 88.2% and a specificity of 64.7% to detect clinical signs of impaired safety of swallow (aspiration or penetration). The test takes 5–10 min to complete. **Discussion and Conclusion:** The V-VST is an excellent tool to screen patients for OD. It combines good psychometric properties, a detailed and easy protocol designed to protect safety of patients, and valid end points to evaluate safety and efficacy of swallowing and detect silent aspirations.

Copyright © 2012 Nestec Ltd., Vevey/S. Karger AG, Basel

Introduction

Oropharyngeal dysphagia (OD) is a major complaint among many patients with neurological diseases and in the elderly, but is not always systematically explored and detected. OD is specifically classified by the World Health Organization in the International Statistical Classification of Diseases and Related Health Problems ICD-9 and ICD-10 (787.2, R13) [1]. Although sufferers are sometimes unaware of their oropharyngeal dysfunction, OD is a highly prevalent clinical condition as it affects more than 30% of patients with stroke, 60–80% of patients with neurodegenerative diseases, up to 13% adults aged 65 and older and more than 51% of institutionalized elderly patients [2, 3]. A Council of Europe resolution claimed that undernutrition among hospital patients is highly prevalent and leads to extended hospital stays, prolonged rehabilitation, and diminished quality of life, and identified OD as a major contributor to malnutrition [4].

Videofluoroscopy (VFS) is the gold standard to study oral and pharyngeal mechanisms of dysphagia and aspiration [5]. However, it is unfeasible to perform a VFS on every patient at risk or with suspected dysphagia. Clinical screening methods with high diagnostic accuracy must be developed to recognize and follow up patients with OD to identify patients who are at risk of aspiration or malnutrition, to identify patients who should be referred for a VFS to assess swallow function, and to help select the most appropriate bolus volume and viscosity for those patients (such as elderly patients admitted to nursing homes) who cannot easily undergo VFS [6]. The volume-viscosity swallow test (V-VST) is a bedside method to screen patients for dysphagia, to identify clinical signs of impaired efficacy and safety of swallow, and to select the appropriate bolus volume and viscosity to achieve the highest safety and efficacy of deglutition [7]. The V-VST method has been designed to favor diagnostic sensitivity as the cost of a false-negative diagnosis of a patient with aspirations is high (aspiration pneumonia) and the cost of a false-positive clinical diagnosis of impaired swallow is low (an unnecessary VFS study). In the validation study of the V-VST, we found a sensitivity and specificity for clinical signs of impaired safety of swallow (aspiration or penetration) of 88.2 and 64.7%, respectively, and a sensitivity of 100% in recognizing patients with aspiration subsequently confirmed by VFS [7].

We have validated the diagnostic accuracy of the V-VST, and we have used it to assess the prevalence of dysphagia among independently living older patients and among patients admitted to our hospital with stroke. The aim of this review is to describe the technique of the V-VST and our experience with this method in the screening of these different phenotypes of patients at risk of OD.

Methods

Management of Oropharyngeal Dysphagia in a General Hospital
The algorithm of management of OD at the Hospital de Mataró (Barcelona, Spain) begins with the identification by a doctor or a nurse of a patient in the risk population for OD, the screening of the nutritional state of the patient by a dietitian, the screening for OD and aspiration by a speech-swallow therapist or trained general practitioner and nurse using the V-VST, and finally, if the result of this process is positive, a videofluoroscopic study of swallow to diagnose the patient, to assess the safety and efficacy of deglutition and to select the treatment for the patient.

Performance of the V-VST

The patient should be sitting, with his back resting against the seatback and feet on the ground. Some pillows can be used to keep the patient in the right position. Hyperextension of the neck should be avoided. The explorer should be placed in front of the patient, sitting slightly below the patient. The explorer will offer the bolus to the patient carefully with a syringe. The exploration (including oxygen saturation measurements) can be recorded with a digital video camera for objective review.

Signs of Impaired Efficacy of Swallow

Efficacy of swallow is evaluated by the identification of the following clinical signs: the efficacy of labial seal, the presence of oral or pharyngeal residue and the presence of piecemeal deglutition (multiple swallows per bolus). The efficacy of labial seal is evaluated by observing if part of the bolus, once placed inside the mouth, escapes through the lips; the presence of oral residue is detected by asking the patient to open his/her mouth after deglutition and observing if part of the bolus remains in the mouth; the presence of pharyngeal residue is detected by asking the patient if he feels some kind of residue or nuisance in the pharynx or the need to swallow another time.

Signs of Impaired Safety of Swallow

Safety of swallow is assessed by evaluating the presence of voice changes, cough or a decrease in oxygen saturation $\geq 3\%$ measured with a finger pulse-oximeter (Nellcor OxiMax, Philips Medical Systems, The Netherlands) placed on the index finger of the right hand. The fall in oxygen saturation is determined by the difference between baseline (baseline readings are obtained 2 min prior to starting the test) and minimum readings during the 2 min period after each swallow. A fall in oxygen saturation $\geq 3\%$ is considered a sign of aspiration into the airway. Before the start of the test, the patient is invited to clearly pronounce his name (or some automatic answer) to obtain the normal pattern of voice. After each deglutition, the patient is invited again to pronounce his name to evaluate if any change is produced. Wet voice, low intensity, lack of voice or the need to clear the throat indicate impaired safety of swallow. The decrease in oxygen saturation and cough can occur before deglutition (indicating the inefficacy of the glossopalatal seal), during deglutition (indicating a delay in the laryngeal vestibule closure) or after deglutition (indicating the presence of residue and a postdeglutitive aspiration).

V-VST Algorithms
Short Algorithm

The volume-viscosity method was designed as an effort test in which boluses of increasing volume and difficulty are administered (fig. 1). The V-VST examines whether patients' swallow efficacy and safety is changed by increasing viscosity. The V-VST was designed to protect patients from aspiration by starting with nectar viscosity and increasing volumes from 5- to 10- and 20-ml boluses in a progression of increasing difficulty. If patients complete the nectar series without major symptoms of aspiration (cough and/or fall in oxygen saturation $\geq 3\%$), a less safe liquid viscosity series is assessed also with boluses of increasing difficulty (5, 10, 20 ml). Finally, a safer pudding viscosity series (5, 10, 20 ml) is assessed in the same way. If the patient presents signs of impaired safety at nectar viscosity, the series is interrupted, the liquid series is omitted and a safer pudding

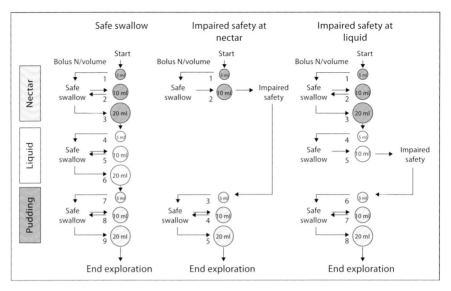

Fig. 1. V-VST short algorithm. Left diagram: patients with safe swallow completed the pathway. Middle diagram: representative pathway for patients with impaired safety at 10 ml nectar. Right diagram: representative pathway for patients with impaired safety at 10 ml liquid.

viscosity series is assessed, and if the pudding viscosity is safe and no residue is observed, pudding viscosity is recommended. If the patient presented signs of impaired safety at liquid viscosity, the liquid series is interrupted and the pudding series is assessed. In this case, the most effective volume of nectar viscosity is recommended.

Long Algorithm

Two additional viscosities can be added at the end of the short algorithm of the V-VST to evaluate the minimum amount of thickener needed to allow a safe and effective swallow. If the patient presents signs of impaired safety at nectar viscosity and the extreme spoon-thick viscosity is safe, a conservative spoon-thick series is assessed. If the patient presents signs of impaired safety at this viscosity, the exploration is interrupted and the extreme spoon-thick viscosity recommended, but if the patient completes the conservative spoon-thick series without major symptoms of aspiration, the honey viscosity is finally evaluated (fig. 2). The aim of the inclusion of these new two viscosity series is to optimize the viscosity needed and to enhance the compliance with the thickener treatment.

Viscosities

The short algorithm of V-VST was validated using a starch-based thickener (Resource ThickenUp, Nestlé Nutrition, Switzerland). The terms used, the amount of thickener necessary to add to 100 ml of water, viscosities obtained, and equivalences with the National Dysphagia Diet Task Force viscosities are shown in table 1. Moreover, the new generation of thickeners based on xanthan gum (Resource ThickenUp Clear, Nestlé Nutrition, Switzerland), can also be used to perform the V-VST; the necessary amount of thickener

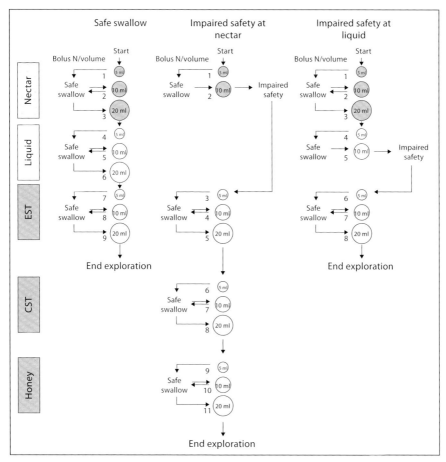

Fig. 2. V-VST long algorithm. Left diagram: patients with safe swallow completed the pathway. Middle diagram: representative pathway for patients with impaired safety at 10 ml nectar and safe swallow at EST viscosity. Right diagram: representative pathway for patients with impaired safety at 10 ml liquid. EST = Extreme spoon-thick; CST = conservative spoon-thick.

to develop the long V-VST algorithm, the viscosities obtained and equivalences with the National Dysphagia Diet Task Force viscosities are also shown in table 1.

Results

In the initial publication of the V-VST [7], 85 patients with OD were evaluated. The etiology of dysphagia of the patients studied was representative of the patients referred for a swallow study and included patients with neurological diseases, patients with neuromuscular degenerative diseases and patients with

Table 1. Equivalences with the National Dysphagia Diet Task Force viscosities, terms, quantity of thickeners and viscosities used in the short and long algorithms of the V-VST

National Dysphagia Diet Task Force		V-VST	Resource ThickenUp		Resource ThickenUp Clear	
	Viscosity mPa s		quantity g/100 ml water	viscosity mPa s	quantity g/100 ml water	viscosity mPa s
Thin	1–50	Liquid	0	21	0	21
Nectar-like	51–350	Nectar	4.5	295	1.2	238
Honey-like	351–1,750	Honey	ND	ND	2.4	766
		Conservative spoon-thick	ND	ND	3.6	1,098
Spoon-thick	>1,750	Extreme spoon-thick	ND	ND	6	1,840
		Pudding	9	3,682	ND	ND

ND = Not determined.

head and neck diseases, including head and neck cancer, Zencker diverticulum and cricopharyngeal bars. Mean duration of clinical assessment of dysphagia by the V-VST was 5.54 ± 2.18 min. By means of the V-VST, the efficacy of swallow was evaluated, and we detected that at liquid viscosity, 4.7% of patients studied presented impaired lip closure, 15.3% piecemeal deglutition, 3.5% oral residue, and 15.3% pharyngeal residue. We also observed that with increased bolus volume and viscosity, the prevalence of piecemeal deglutition and oral and pharyngeal residue was increased. Safety of swallow was also assessed, and we detected that 50% of patients presented clinical signs of impaired safety of swallow (cough, changes in voice or a fall in oxygen saturation ≥3%) during 5-ml liquid bolus. In this study, up to 48% of patients with aspirations at VFS did not present cough (silent aspirators) and were clinically recognized by the V-VST by a fall in oxygen saturation ≥3% and/or changes in voice after swallow. By means of the V-VST, we found that safety of swallow was significantly reduced by bolus volume and improved by increasing bolus viscosity. We also found in this study that the probability of a therapeutic effect (positive predictive value) from increasing viscosity to reduce penetrations and aspirations in patients identified by the V-VST was 98.9%.

The V-VST was also used to assess the prevalence of OD in independently living older persons (>70 years) [8]. Authors found that 27.2% of the 254 persons recruited presented signs of OD, 20.5% presented signs of impaired efficacy of swallow, and 15.4%, signs of impaired safety of swallow. The sensitivity and specificity of the test were used to estimate the prevalence of dysphagia in this population. The systematic application of the V-VST was also used to manage patients admitted with acute stroke to the neurology unit of the Hospital de Mataró [9]. We evaluated 98 consecutively admitted patients with the V-VST and found 60 (61.2%) presented signs of OD, 18.6% of the dysphagic patients presented signs of impaired safety of swallow, 20.3% signs of impaired efficacy, and 61.1% of them, both. Results of the V-VST were used to introduce compensatory dietary strategies based on the adaptation of viscosity and consistency of fluids and solids, to identify patients and risk of malnutrition (as dysphagia is a recognized cause of malnutrition in these patients), and to refer patients to speech language pathologists or to dietitians when appropriate to modify patients' diets, to make new assessments of swallow function if necessary, and to educate patients and caregivers about the dysphagia diet [9].

Discussion

The V-VST is a bedside screening method by which boluses of different volumes and viscosities are administered quickly, safely and accurately to screen for dysphagia in hospitalized and independently living patients with multiple etiologies. Moreover, the V-VST systematically evaluates clinical signs of safety and efficacy of swallow and detects patients with silent aspirations. The V-VST identifies patients who need further exploration by VFS and helps to select the ideal bolus volume and viscosity for liquids when a VFS study cannot be performed. The V-VST can be administered by any member of the multidisciplinary dysphagia team, facilitating the screening of dysphagia at all medical facilities and at any time of day, and can be repeated according the natural progression of the disease.

Previous to the publication of the V-VST method, Bours et al. [10] carried out a systematic review of the effectiveness and feasibility of bedside screening methods in detecting dysphagia in patients with neurological disorders. A form with nine items evaluating the validity, generalizability and reliability of studies was used to assess the methodological quality of the published studies, and 11 of them were considered to have sufficient quality. Using the same assessment, the V-VST study can also be classified as a study with 'good methodological quality' because just one item was not satisfied, item 2, as patients studied in the validation study of the VVST were referred for evaluation because they presented swallowing difficulties (table 2). Bours et al. [10], in their systematic review, recommend a water test combined with oximetry using coughing, choking and

Table 2. Items for the methodological assessment of the quality of studies assessing the quality of bedside screening tests for evaluation of swallowing

1. Were the reference test and the index test interpreted independently (blind)?	Yes
2. Was the index test applied independent of relevant information on clinical data of the patient regarding the target condition?	No
3. Was the reference test applied to all patients who received the index test?	Yes
4. Was the period between the reference test and the index test short enough to be reasonably sure that the target condition did not change between the two tests? (within 24 h in acute stroke, and within 7 days in other neurological diseases)	Yes
5. Was the selection of the study population valid?	Yes
6. Are data presented in enough detail to calculate appropriate test characteristics?	Yes
7. Was the study population appropriate to evaluate the proposed use of the index test?	Yes
8. Was the index test described in detail so it could be reproduced?	Yes
9. Were adequate definitions used for normal/abnormal reference test results and normal/abnormal index test results?	Yes

Adapted from Bours et al. [10]. Results of the evaluation of the V-VST.

voice alteration as the end points as the best method to screen patients for dysphagia. The water tests belong to the most extended and frequently used tests for dysphagia screening. They presented a sensitivity of 51–85% and a specificity of 66–75% to detect aspirations, and a sensitivity of 27–79% and specificity of 63–88% to detect impaired safety of swallow (penetrations or aspirations) [11–13]. These parameters are similar to the V-VST, but the water tests involve the continuous swallow of large amounts of water which may place the patient at risk of aspiration. Moreover, aspirations that occur without any clinical manifestation (silent aspirations) cannot be detected by water tests alone. This parameter is resolved with the combination of the water test with the monitoring of oxygen desaturation [14, 15]. However, the water tests do not assess any parameter related to the efficacy of swallow or evaluate the ability of patients to swallow different viscosities.

Like the V-VST, several tests have been developed using different viscosities and solids to evaluate aspiration and/or penetration. Sensitivity of these trials ranges from 41 to 100% and specificity from 57 to 82% [16–18]. Although these tests evaluate patients' ability to swallow material of different consistencies, if they are not combined with oxygen desaturation, silent aspirations can be lost.

Finally, Smith et al. [19] recommended a water test combined with oxygen saturation followed by bedside swallowing assessment with a variety of quantities and consistencies. This protocol showed a sensitivity of 80% and specificity of 68%, but the authors did not provide a detailed protocol for the swallow test and only acute poststroke patients were studied.

Conclusion

The V-VST combines good psychometric properties, feasibility, a detailed and easy to perform protocol, an algorithm designed to protect patients' safety, enough end points to evaluate the safety and efficacy of swallowing, and a system to detect silent aspirations. The V-VST detects patients who need a diagnostic study (VFS or FEES) or dietary modifications when the VFS study is not possible. We believe that the V-VST is an excellent clinical tool to screen patients for dysphagia. Patients with a positive test should undergo VFS for a full assessment of swallow function.

References

1 International Statistical Classification of Diseases and Related Health Problems. http://apps.who.int/classifications/apps/icd/icd10online/?gr10.htm±r13, accessed July 21, 2011.
2 Turley R, Cohen S: Impact of voice and swallowing problems in the elderly. Otolaryngol Head Neck Surg 2009;140:33–36.
3 Lin LC, Wu SC, Chen HS, et al: Prevalence of impaired swallowing in institutionalized older people in Taiwan. J Am Geriatr Soc 2002;50:1118–1123.
4 Resolution ResAP(2003)3 on food and nutritional care in hospitals. 860th meeting of the Ministers' Deputies. Council of Europe, Committee of Ministers. https://wcd.coe.int/wcd/ViewDoc.jsp?Ref=ResAP(2003)3&Language=lanEnglish&Site=CM&BackColorInternet=C3C3C3&BackColorIntranet=EDB021&BackColorLogged=F5D383, accessed July 21, 2011.
5 Cook IJ, Kahrilas PJ: AGA technical review on management of oropharyngeal dysphagia. Gastroenterology 1999;116:455–478.
6 Connolly MJ: Of proverbs and prevention: aspiration and its consequences in older patients. Age Ageing 2010;39:2–4.
7 Clave P, Arreola V, Romea M, et al: Accuracy of the volume-viscosity swallow test for clinical screening of oropharyngeal dysphagia and aspiration. Clin Nutr 2008;27:806–815.
8 Serra-Prat M, Hinojosa G, Lopez D, et al: Prevalence of oropharyngeal dysphagia and impaired safety and efficacy of swallow in independently living older persons. J Am Geriatr Soc 2011;59:186–187.

9 Sebastián ML, Palomeras E, Clave P, et al: La disfágia en el ictus agudo: actuaciones de Enfermeria. Rev Cien Soc Esp Enferm Neurol 2009;29:8–11.
10 Bours GJ, Speyer R, Lemmens J, et al: Bedside screening tests vs. videofluoroscopy or fibreoptic endoscopic evaluation of swallowing to detect dysphagia in patients with neurological disorders: systematic review. J Adv Nurs 2009;65:477–493.
11 Daniels SK, McAdam CP, Brailey K, et al: Clinical Assessment of swallowing and prediction of dysphagia severity. Am J Speech Lang Pathol 2011;6:17–24.
12 Mari F, Matei M, Ceravolo MG, et al: Predictive value of clinical indices in detecting aspiration in patients with neurological disorders. J Neurol Neurosurg Psychiatry 1997;63:456–460.
13 Smithard DG, O'Neill PA, Park C, et al: Can bedside assessment reliably exclude aspiration following acute stroke? Age Ageing 1998;27:99–106.
14 Lim SH, Lieu PK, Phua SY, et al: Accuracy of bedside clinical methods compared with fiberoptic endoscopic examination of swallowing (FEES) in determining the risk of aspiration in acute stroke patients. Dysphagia 2001;16:1–6.
15 Chong MS, Lieu PK, Sitoh YY, et al: Bedside clinical methods useful as screening test for aspiration in elderly patients with recent and previous strokes. Ann Acad Med Singapore 2003;32:790–794.

16   Logemann JA, Veis S, Colangelo L: A screen-
     ing procedure for oropharyngeal dysphagia.
     Dysphagia 1999;14:44–51.
17   McCullough GH, Wertz RT, Rosenbek JC:
     Sensitivity and specificity of clinical/bedside
     examination signs for detecting aspiration
     in adults subsequent to stroke. J Commun
     Disord 2001;34:55–72.

18   Trapl M, Enderle P, Nowotny M, et al:
     Dysphagia bedside screening for acute-stroke
     patients: the Gugging Swallowing Screen.
     Stroke 2007;38:2948–2952.
19   Smith HA, Lee SH, O'Neill PA, et al: The
     combination of bedside swallowing assess-
     ment and oxygen saturation monitor-
     ing of swallowing in acute stroke: a safe
     and humane screening tool. Age Ageing
     2000;29:495–499.

Cichero J, Clavé P (eds): Stepping Stones to Living Well with Dysphagia.
Nestlé Nutr Inst Workshop Ser, vol 72, pp 43–52,
Nestec Ltd., Vevey/S. Karger AG., Basel, © 2012

Videofluoroscopic Swallow Study: Techniques, Signs and Reports

Margareta Bülow

Diagnostic Centre of Imaging and Functional Medicine, Skåne University Hospital Malmö, Malmö, Sweden

Abstract

Management of oropharyngeal swallowing dysfunction often requires both a clinical and an instrumental examination. A videofluoroscopic swallowing study is an instrumental examination that often could be a good option and a very useful tool for the swallowing clinician. At Skåne University Hospital, Malmö, Sweden, the name of such examination is therapeutic videoradiographic swallowing study (TVSS). A TVSS examination should always be performed in collaboration between a speech language pathologist and a radiologist. During the examination, the patient is seated in an upright position, but the examination can also be performed with the patient lying down. The TVSS examination can be performed both in frontal and lateral projection. Test material with varied consistencies as well as different therapeutic strategies can be tested during the examination. Any oral and/or pharyngeal dysfunction can be defined, for example a delay in the initiation of the pharyngeal swallow or an absent pharyngeal swallow, pharyngeal retention, penetration, and silent aspiration. After the examination, an analysis is performed, and it is studied how different textures affect the physiology of swallowing. A report is then written in which the actual dysfunction is described in detail, and recommendations regarding modified textures and swallowing techniques are given.

Introduction

In the management of oropharyngeal swallowing dysfunction, both clinical and instrumental swallowing examinations may be necessary. Clinical experience and research findings provide evidence that aspiration, and more importantly the cause of aspiration, can be missed during observations made from test swallows included in a clinical or bedside examination [1].

The instrumental technique has to be chosen based on what the clinician wants to know to be able to take decisions regarding appropriate therapeutic management. At the Diagnostic Centre of Imaging and Functional Medicine, Skåne University Hospital, Malmö, Sweden, radiology has for many years been the first-choice instrumental technique to examine oropharyngeal swallowing problems. We differentiate between two radiological swallowing examinations. One is the more traditional hypopharynx-esophagus examination with focus on morphologic aspects. The other one is the videofluoroscopic swallowing examination with focus on swallowing function, and at our hospital it is named therapeutic videoradiographic swallowing study (TVSS). The therapeutic swallowing study is a dynamic procedure, and the mechanical passage of food and liquid with varied textures and viscosity can be followed from the mouth to the stomach. For a comprehensive examination, observation of oral bolus manipulation, lingual motility efficiency of mastication, timing of pharyngeal swallow initiation, soft palate elevation and retraction, tongue base retraction, pharyngeal contraction, superior and anterior hyolaryngeal movement, epiglottic inversion and extent and duration of pharyngoesophageal segment opening have to be observed. Also therapeutic strategies can be tested during such swallowing examinations, and their effect on the swallowing physiology analyzed [2–11]. The TVSS examination should always be performed in collaboration between a speech language pathologist (SLP) and a radiologist. The combination of the expertise of the two professionals makes the examination an excellent diagnostic tool (fig. 1).

Equipment

To perform a TVSS examination, a laboratory with radiologic fluoroscopic equipment is required. Recording and storage of the examination require a computer disc or videotape that makes it possible to analyze structural movements in relation to contrast flow in slow motion and frame by frame after the examination. However, in most radiological settings, digital radiography is nowadays used, and for storage different high-resolution videofluoroscopic digital recording devices are used. Afterwards, the examination can be transmitted digitally to an electronic picture archiving and communication system. Such techniques are easy to handle, provide rapid retrieval, and the availability is excellent. Any pathophysiology can be analyzed in detail related to the flow of the given textures. Disordered timing and coordination of structural movement as well as the presence, degree, timing and cause of aspiration can be documented.

The examination can be performed using minimal radiation doses. In a study from the UK, the authors found that the radiation doses were 0.2 mSv dose area for the average videofluoroscopic examination [12]. From our clinical experience, we have found that the radiation exposure time in the average case is 2–3 min (fig. 2).

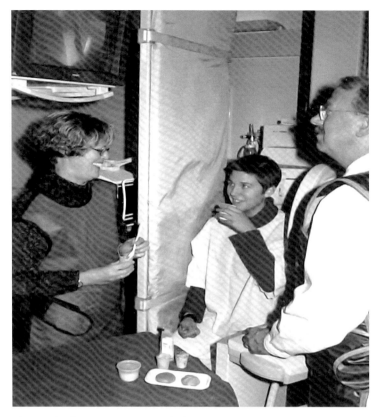

Fig. 1. The fluoroscopy suite with the SLP, the radiologist, and the patient prepared for a swallowing examination in lateral projection.

The Procedure

To be able to perform a TVSS examination, and for an accurate and reliable implementation and interpretation of test results, specialized training for both the SLP and the radiologist is required [13].

At our hospital, the SLP has her own schedule at the laboratory and has the opportunity to schedule 8 patients every week. This makes the availability to the radiology suite easier, and the patient can often be scheduled for the examination within short time, and sometimes if necessary the same day the clinical examination has been performed.

During the examination, the radiologist operates the fluoroscopic equipment and observes anatomic abnormalities. The SLP takes decides how to perform the examination often based on observations of the patient during a bedside examination. The assistant nurse feeds the patient. If possible, the patients feed themselves, which gives important information about their habitual eating and drinking behaviors.

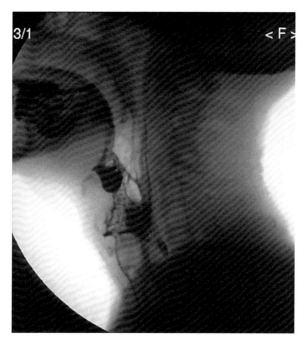

Fig. 2. Patient positioned in lateral view during a videofluoroscopic swallowing examination. A severe dysfunction can be seen with both aspiration to the trachea, and pharyngeal residue.

Focus during the TVSS examination is on the oral and the pharyngeal phases of swallowing. Most often, the study begins with the subject positioned in lateral view, the optimal position for visualizing penetration or aspiration of material into the laryngeal vestibule before, during, and after swallowing. The profile contours of the soft palate, base of the tongue, posterior pharyngeal wall, epiglottis, aryepiglottic folds, anterior hypo-pharyngeal wall and the region of the cricopharyngeal muscle or pharyngoesophageal segment can be observed in the lateral view. If necessary, the patient is then positioned in a frontal view permitting observation regarding asymmetric contours, the surface of the base of the tongue, median and lateral glossoepiglottic folds, tonsillar fossa, valleculae and hypopharynx.

In most cases, the patient is seated in an upright position, but if necessary it is also possible to perform the examination with the patient lying down. Fixed routines are used, but it is also possible, if necessary, with an individually adapted examination (table 1).

Different textures are given to the patient to identify optimal food and liquid that facilitates a safe and efficient oral intake. Every patient has to be given his or her individual combination of test material depending on the nature of the swallowing problem.

Bülow

Table 1. Routines during the examination

Radiologist	Operates the fluoroscopic equipment
	Observes anatomic abnormalities
	Analyzes the exam together with the SLP
SLP	Makes decisions about how to perform the procedure, often based on a clinical examination
	Completes the swallowing protocol
	Analyzes the exam together with the radiologist
	Writes the report
Assistant nurse	Prepares the fluoroscopy suite for examination
	Assists the patient before and after the procedure
	Prepares the test material
	Feeds the patient

In our research, we have found that carbonated liquids can be a good option to improve swallowing for many of our patients, and such liquids are therefore included in our routine protocol. It is, however, of importance that the liquid has been individually tested before being prescribed [14]. Also, cold sour texture may be a good option for several dysphagic patients [15].

Sometimes, it could be observed that oral nutrition is not possible due to a severe swallowing dysfunction. In such cases, tube feeding may be regarded as the only safe and efficient option for feeding. However, sometimes the patient could have tube feedings as the primary source of nutrition and hydration, combined with safe supplementation of small amounts of modified food and liquid textures for pleasure and optimization of quality of life.

The test material is prepared according to our recipe, composed after many years of clinical experience and collaboration with a dietician. The test material is mixed with barium contrast in the hospital kitchen, with assistance from a nurse from the radiological department. Our test materials are prepared from ordinary food that makes it easy to recognize and is thereby familiar to our patients. The ready-made textures are sent to the radiological department in small cans, 0.5 dl for a solid bolus and 1 dl for liquids. They are placed in a freezer until needed. The test material has to be dense enough to allow X-ray visualization. Barium sulphate is often used that allows for optimal visualization of bolus passage through the alimentary tract [16]. However, it has been found that sensory properties of food may be affected by adding barium sulphate [17–19]. So, even if the sensory properties of the test food may be affected by adding barium sulphate, we have also learned from clinical experience from thousands of examinations that it is possible to define the nature of the actual dysfunction in a reliable way. That makes it possible to take decisions regarding most appropriate therapeutic strategies,

Table 2. Different textures used at the TVSS examination

Solids	Pudding
	Timbale
	Paté
	Chopped normal food
	(sour cold sorbet)
Liquids	Thickened liquid
	Carbonated liquid
	Thin liquid
Patient brings own material	

and modified textures, and thereby guide the patient to a safe and efficient swallowing.

During the examination, controlled amounts of food and liquid textures are administered to the patient. We always start the examination with small amounts of pudding or thickened liquid consistencies (3 ml and then go further with 5, 10 ml or more). If possible, each consistency is given twice. Also free drinking is tested since that can give valuable information about the amount the patient takes and how the specific liquid is handled. The patients may, if possible, also feed themselves. The patient can also, if he or she reports symptoms with only very specific food or liquid items, bring own material to the examination where it will be mixed with barium contrast and tested. If we suspect aspiration and/ or if we do not know for sure whether the patient will initiate a pharyngeal swallow or not, the procedure starts with 2 or 3 ml of water-soluble contrast either as thin or thickened liquid. The patient should not be exposed to any risks of aspiration and its complications (table 2).

For a comprehensive examination, observation of oral bolus manipulation, lingual motility, efficiency of mastication, timing of pharyngeal swallow initiation, soft palate elevation and retraction, tongue base retraction, pharyngeal contraction, superior and anterior hyolaryngeal movement, epiglottic inversion and extent and duration of pharyngoesophageal segment opening must be included [7]. It is also of importance to follow at least one or two swallows through the esophagus to identify a free passage. If any esophageal dysfunction is suspected, the patient will be recommended further examinations and referred to appropriate professionals (table 3).

Also different therapeutic techniques may, if necessary, systematically be applied based on the observed nature of the swallowing disorder. Such techniques include postural techniques, maneuvers and techniques improving oral sensory awareness, and their effect on function can be observed during the examination [20–27]. When testing different swallowing techniques during the

Table 3. Swallowing physiology and dysfunction

Oral-phase physiology	Oral dysfunction
Lip closure	Aspiration before pharyngeal swallow
Texture preparation	Leakage (anterior, posterior)
Tongue movements	Oral residue
Mastication	Inefficient tongue movements and mastication
Bolus transport	Delayed bolus transport
Closure into nasal cavity	Diffuse spreading of bolus in oral cavity
	Lingual propulsion of food and liquid
	Regurgitation into nasal cavity
Pharyngeal-phase physiology	**Pharyngeal dysfunction**
Laryngeal elevation	Aspiration during swallow
Hyoid bone movement	Reduced laryngeal elevation
Epiglottic tilt	Incomplete movements of the hyoid bone
Vestibulum laryngis closure	Incomplete epiglottic closure
Vestibulum laryngis closure:	Vestibulum laryngis:
penetration/aspiration	subepiglottic penetration
Constrictor muscle activity:	supraglottic penetration
pharyngeal retention	tracheal penetration/aspiration
	Delayed initiation of pharyngeal swallow
	Absent pharyngeal swallow
Pharyngoesophageal segment (PES) opening	
Esophageal-phase physiology	**Esophageal dysfunction**
PES opening	Incomplete/absent PES opening
	Regurgitation from esophagus to pyriform sinuses
	Incomplete peristalsis
	Strictures

TVSS examination, it is important to be aware of the fact that it could be difficult for the patient to perform a special technique just after a short instruction. Most often, a period of training is required to be able to perform the different techniques properly. In our research, we found that even if the patients could not perform a single technique quite properly during videofluoroscopy, they got an increased knowledge and awareness about how to swallow in a safe way, and that resulted in an improved concentration when they swallowed, and thereby we saw fewer misdirected swallows [24].

Of importance is that caregivers, nurses (e.g. depending on the medical status of the patient) and/or family members have the opportunity to observe the study. Most efficient at the time of the examination but also a later viewing of the recorded examination is possible. Such information makes it possible to educate the caregivers about the nature of the patient's swallowing problem. Necessary precautions and management strategies that must be applied to ensure airway protection and efficient oral intake can be explained.

Analyses and Report

To analyze and to document the examination, different types of protocols are used [28, 29]. Both quantitative and qualitative measuring can be done. The Rosenbek penetration-aspiration scale [30] is a well-known and an often used measuring scale. Several swallowing clinics have developed their own protocol. At our Department, we have protocols for both quantitative and qualitative analyses.

After the examination, the SLP and the radiologist together analyze the entire examination and study how different textures and therapeutic strategies affect the physiology of swallowing. Decisions regarding an appropriate management plan are discussed. After that, a report is written in which the actual pathophysiology is explained in detail, recommendations are given including the safest nutrition and involves in most cases a texture-modified diet and if necessary also different therapeutic strategies. Sometimes a TVSS examination does not give enough information regarding actual problems, and the patient has to be referred for further examinations; for example, a contact with a gastroenterologist, neurologist or an ENT-specialist may be necessary.

Conclusion

A TVSS examination should be performed in collaboration between a SLP and a radiologist. Focus during the examination is on the oral and the pharyngeal phases of the swallowing sequence. Different textures as well as different therapeutic strategies can be tested during the examination. Any swallowing dysfunction shows individual characterization, and therefore recommendations regarding a safe and efficient nutrition have to be based on the individuals' actual pathophysiology. Either modified textures or if necessary tube feeding and/or different therapeutic strategies can be prescribed.

References

1 Splaingard ML, Hutchins B, Sulton LD, Chauhuri G: Aspiration in rehabilitation patients: videofluoroscopy vs. bedside clinical assessment. Arch Phys Med Rehabil 1988;69:637–640.

2 Logemann JA: A manual for the videofluoroscopic evaluation of swallowing. Boston, College-Hill Press, 1986.

3 Donner M: The evaluation of dysphagia by radiography and other methods of imaging. Dysphagia 1988;1:49–50.

4 Dodds WJ, Logemann JA, Stewart ET: Radiological assessment of abnormal oral and pharyngeal phases of swallow. AJR Am J Roentgenol 1990;154:965–974.

5 Dodds WJ, Stewart ET, Logemann J: Physiology and radiology of the normal oral and pharyngeal phases of swallowing. AJR Am J Roentgenol 1990;154:993–963.

6 Ekberg O: The role of radiology in evaluation and treatment of neurologically-impaired patients with dysphagia. J Neurol Rehabil 1990;4:65–73.

7 Ekberg O: Radiologic evaluation of swallowing; in Groher ME (ed): Dysphagia. Diagnosis and Management, ed 2. Boston, Butterworth-Heineman, 1992, pp 163–195.

8 Martin-Harris B, Logemann JA, McMahon S, et al: Clinical utility of the modified barium swallow. Dysphagia 2000;15:136–141.

9 Bülow M, Martin Harris B: The therapeutic swallowing study; in Ekberg O (ed): Radiology of the Pharynx and the Esophagus. Berlin, Springer, 2003, pp 99–108.

10 Gates J, Hartnell GG, Graminga GD: Videofluoroscopy and swallowing studies for neurologc disease: a primer. Radiographics 2006;26:e22.

11 Martin-Harris B, Jones B: The videofluorographic swallowing study. Phys Med Rehabil Clin N Am 2008;19:769–785.

12 Zammit-Maempel I, Chapple C-L, Leslie P: Radiation dose in videofluoroscopic swallow studies. Dysphagia 2007;22:13–15.

13 Logemann JA, Lazarus CL, Phillips Keely S, et al: Effectiveness of four hours of education in interpretation of radiographic studies. Dysphagia 2000;15:180–183.

14 Bülow M, Olsson R, Ekberg O: Videoradiographic analysis of how carbonated thin thickened liquids affect the physiology of swallowing in subjects with aspiration on thin liquids. Acta Radiol 2003;44:366–372.

15 Cola PC, Gatto AR, Silva RG, et al: The influence of sour taste and cold temperature in pharyngeal transit duration in patients with stroke. Arq Gastroenterol 2010;47:18–21.

16 Murray J: Videofluoroscopic examination; in Murray J (ed): Manual of Dysphagia Assessment in Adults. San Diego, Singular Publishing Group, 1999, chapter 3, pp 113–151.

17 Groher ME, Crary MA, Carnaby Mann G, et al: The impact of rheologically controlled materials on the identifications of airway compromise on the clinical and videofluoroscopic swallowing examinations. Dysphagia 2006;21:218–225.

18 Ekberg O, Bülow M, Ekman S, et al: Effect of barium sulphate contrast medium on rheology and sensory texture attributes in a model food. Acta Radiol 2009;50:131–138.

19 Wendin K, Ekman S, Bülow M, et al: Objective and quantitative definitions of modified food textures based on sensory and rheological methodology. Food Nutr Res DOI: 10.3402/fnr.v54i0.5134.

20 Ekberg O: Posture of the head and pharyngeal swallow. Acta Radiol Diagn 1986;27:691–696.

21 Logemann J: Evaluation and Treatment of Swallowing Disorders. Austin, Pro-Ed, 1998.

22 Bülow M, Olsson R, Ekberg O: Videomanometric analysis of supraglottic swallow, effortful swallow and chin tuck in healthy volunteers. Dysphagia 1999;14:67–72.

23 Bülow M, Olsson R, Ekberg O: Videomanometric analysis of supraglottic swallow, effortful swallow and chin tuck in patients with pharyngeal dysfunction. Dysphagia 2001;16:190–195.

24 Bülow M: Therapeutic aspects of oral and pharyngeal swallowing dysfunction. Videoradiographic and videomanometric analyses of adult healthy volunteers and dysphagic patients; thesis, Lund University, 2003.

25 Logemann JA: Treatment of oral and pharyngeal dysphagia. Phys Med Rehabil Clin N Am 2008;19:803 816, ix.

26 Bodén K, Hallgren A, Witt Hedström H: Effects of three swallow maneuvers analyzed by videomanometry. Acta Radiol 2006;47:628–633.

27 Baylow HE, Goldfarb R, Taveira CH, Steinberg RS: Accuracy of clinical judgment of the chin-down posture for dysphagia during the clinical/bedside assessment as corroborated by videofluoroscopy in adults with acute stroke. Dysphagia 2009;24:423–433.

28 Bingjie L, Tong Z, Xinting S, et al: Quantitative videofluoroscopic analysis of penetration-aspiration in post-stroke patients. Neurol India 2010;58:42–47.

29 Van der Kruis JG, Baijens LW, Speyer R, Zwijnenberg I: Biomechanical analysis of hyoid bone displacement in videofluoroscopy: a systematic review of intervention effects. Dysphagia 2011;26:171–182.

30 Rosenbek JC, Robbins J, Roecker EV, et al: A penetration-aspiration scale. Dysphagia 1996;11:93–98.

Cichero J, Clavé P (eds): Stepping Stones to Living Well with Dysphagia.
Nestlé Nutr Inst Workshop Ser, vol 72, pp 53–56,
Nestec Ltd., Vevey/S. Karger AG., Basel, © 2012

Screening and Clinical Assessment of Oropharyngeal Dysphagia

Rosemary Martino

Department of Speech Language Pathology, University of Toronto, Toronto, ON, Canada

Abstract

Dysphagia is common after stroke, and has been associated with serious consequences such as pneumonia, malnutrition, dehydration and even death. There is emerging evidence that early detection with screening may reduce these consequences. As clinicians, it is our responsibility to strive to service our patients with the best evidence and implement screening protocols that are reliable, valid and feasible.

Copyright © 2012 Nestec Ltd., Vevey/S. Karger AG, Basel

Dysphagia is common after stroke, presenting in approximately 55% of all acute hospitalized stroke patients, and depending on the lesion site and volume, can linger as a chronic problem for years afterward [1]. Dysphagia is present when food or liquids are not transported efficiently or safely through the aerodigestive tract. It manifests along a continuum of severity from mild (foods reside in the pharynx after the swallow) to severe (liquids enter the lungs).

Epidemiology of Dysphagia

Dysphagia is not a disease but rather a consequence of existing diseases such as stroke. It is predicted that there will be approximately 15,000–21,000 new stroke patients per year over age 65 with dysphagia in Canada [2], and 200,000 in the US. Of these patients, as many as 10,000 in Canada and 100,000 in the US likely continue to suffer dysphagia for months following their initial stroke event. Assuming no change in current health care interventions and in the direction of aging population demographics [3], the overall economic burden of treating the consequences of dysphagia can be expected to increase dramatically over the next few years.

Consequences of Dysphagia

Dysphagia has been associated with consequences, such as increased length of stay, malnutrition, dehydration and even death [4]. Reports of pneumonia in stroke patients with dysphagia range between 7 and 33%, with conservative estimates at 18% [1]. Stroke patients with dysphagia have a 3-fold increased risk for aspiration pneumonia, and this risk is markedly increased to 11-fold in stroke patients with confirmed aspiration on videofluoroscopy [1]. Aspiration without a cough (silent aspiration) further increases the incidence of pneumonia to 64% [5]. This is problematic considering that silent aspiration occurs in up to two thirds of stroke patients [6]. If left undetected, dysphagia can lead to serious comorbidities.

Swallowing Physiology

To properly diagnose dysphagia, it is important to understand the normal swallowing mechanism. Under normal physiological conditions, humans swallow 1,000–3,000 times daily and significantly less during the night. Swallowing includes not only eating and drinking but also clearing of the esophagus. Normal swallowing involves four sequential phases: oral preparation, oral transport, pharyngeal and esophageal.

Screening Assessment of Dysphagia

The main purpose for clinical screening is to identify patients at risk for oropharyngeal dysphagia and initiate early referral for diagnosis and treatment in order to prevent distressing dysphagia symptoms and to minimize risks for pneumonia, malnutrition and dehydration [2]. In order to have clinical utility, the screening tool must have proven reliability and validity. Psychometrically, a screening tool aims to identify those patients at greatest risk for dysphagia; therefore, it must have high sensitivity [7]. The sensitivity of a test is defined as the proportion of patients with the attribute who are correctly identified by the test, also known as the true positive value [8]. In this way, screening serves to rule out those patients who likely do not have dysphagia.

Bours et al. [9] conducted a systematic review of published screening tools in search for one that is properly standardized. Their findings identified no such screening tool. These authors made a plea for further research to establish the most effective standardized protocol to accurately detect aspiration at the bedside. Several researchers have since answered this plea. In the recent years, there have been several published studies introducing new screening tools. In response to the identified gap in the literature relating to availability of accurate screening tools and an effort to standardize care for stroke patients across all settings, the Toronto Bedside Swallowing Screening Test (TOR-BSST©) was developed [7]. The TOR-BSST© is a brief screening tool that predicts the presence of dysphagia in stroke survivors. Its items were generated using the best available evidence derived from an extensive systematic review [2]. The TOR-BSST© is unique in that it has proven high reliability and validity with stroke patients in both acute and rehabilitation settings. This tool is now being validated with etiologies other than stroke in studies currently underway. Other screening tools that are available in the literature for review include those for patients with Parkinson's disease [10] and mixed etiologies [11–14].

Although a completely satisfactory screening tool has not been available until more recently, there is already evidence for the benefit of screening from multi-site survey research [15]. A lower rate of pneumonia was identified in sites with a formal dysphagia screening program, regardless of screening method utilized, compared to sites with no such screening program. Although these reports of screening benefit to health were a result of screening tools that were not properly standardized, it is logical to assume that the benefits would be even greater with the use of a dysphagia screening tool that has been systematically developed and tested for stability and accuracy. The added practical and economic value of a screening test that accurately rules out dysphagia is obvious.

As clinicians, we strive to service our patients according to the best available evidence. Hence, we need to appraise the new screening tools that are now available to ensure their proper scientific development and psychometric standards. In light of these new tools, it is no longer sufficient to just implement a dysphagia program with any tool, as did Hinchey and colleagues [14], but instead it is our responsibly to ensure that we select the tool that has been developed according to published standards and with a large patient population across the continuum of care and with proven psychometric properties.

References

1 Martino R, Foley N, Bhogal S, et al: Dysphagia after stroke: incidence, diagnosis, and pulmonary complications. Stroke 2005;36:2756–2763.
2 Martino R, Pron G, Diamant NE: Screening for oropharyngeal dysphagia in stroke: insufficient evidence for guidelines. Dysphagia 2000;15:19–30.
3 Statistics Canada. Annual Demographic Statistics, 1994, 1995.
4 Altman KW, Yu GP, Schaefer SD: Consequence of dysphagia in the hospitalized patient: impact on prognosis and hospital resources. Arch Otolaryngol Head Neck Surg 2010;136:784–789.

5   Nakajoh K, Nakagawa T, Sekizawa K, et al: Relation between incidence of pneumonia and protective reflexes in post-stroke patients with oral or tube feeding. J Intern Med 2000;247:39–42.

6   Daniels SK, Brailey K, Priestly DH, et al: Aspiration in patients with acute stroke. Arch Phys Med Rehabil 1998;79:14–19.

7   Martino R, Silver F, Teasell R, et al: The Toronto Bedside Swallowing Screening Test (TOR-BSST©): development and validation of a dysphagia screening tool for patients with stroke. Stroke 2009;40:555–561.

8   Streiner DL: Diagnosing tests: using and misusing diagnostic and screening tests. J Pers Assess 2003;81:209–219.

9   Bours GJ, Speyer R, Lemmens J, et al: Bedside screening tests vs. videofluoroscopy or fibreoptic endoscopic evaluation of swallowing to detect dysphagia in patients with neurological disorders: systematic review. J Adv Nurs 2009;65:477–493.

10 Lam K, Lam FK, Lau KK, et al: Simple clinical tests may predict severe oropharyngeal dysphagia in Parkinson's disease. Mov Disord 2007;22:640–644.

11 Clave P, Arreola V, Romea M, et al: Accuracy of the volume-viscosity swallow test for clinical screening of oropharyngeal dysphagia and aspiration. Clin Nutr 2008;27:806–815.

12 Nathadwarawala KM, Nicklin J, Wiles CM: A timed test of swallowing capacity for neurological patients. J Neurol Neurosurg Psychiatry 1992;55:822–825.

13 Suiter DM, Leder SB: Clinical utility of the 3-ounce water swallow test. Dysphagia 2008;23:244–250.

14 Cichero J, Heaton S, Bassett L: Triaging dysphagia: nurse screening for dysphagia in an acute hospital. J Clin Nurs 2009;18:1649–1659.

15 Hinchey JA, Shephard T, Furie K, et al: Formal dysphagia screening protocols prevent pneumonia. Stroke 2005;36:1972–1976.

Dysfunction and Related Complications

Cichero J, Clavé P (eds): Stepping Stones to Living Well with Dysphagia.
Nestlé Nutr Inst Workshop Ser, vol 72, pp 57–66,
Nestec Ltd., Vevey/S. Karger AG., Basel, © 2012

Pathophysiology, Relevance and Natural History of Oropharyngeal Dysphagia among Older People

Pere Clavé[a,b] · Laia Rofes[b] · Silvia Carrión[a] ·
Omar Ortega[a] · Mateu Cabré[c] · Mateu Serra-Prat[d] ·
Viridiana Arreola[a]

[a]Unitat d'Exploracions Funcionals Digestives, Department of Surgery, Hospital de Mataró, Universitat Autònoma de Barcelona, [b]Centro de Investigación Biomédica en Red, Enfermedades Hepáticas y Digestivas, Insituto de Salud Carlos III, Ministerio de Sanidad y Consumo, [c]Unidad Geriátirca de Agudos and [d]Unitat de Recerca, Hospital de Mataró, Barcelona, Spain

Abstract

Oropharyngeal dysphagia (OD) is a very frequent condition among older people with a prevalence ranging from mild symptoms in 25% of the independently living to severe symptoms in more than 50% living in nursing homes. There are several validated methods of screening, and clinical assessment and videofluoroscopy are the gold standard for the study of the mechanisms of OD in the elderly. Oropharyngeal residue is mainly caused by weak bolus propulsion forces due to tongue sarcopenia. The neural elements of swallow response are also impaired in older persons, with prolonged and delayed laryngeal vestibule closure and slow hyoid movement causing oropharyngeal aspirations. OD causes malnutrition, dehydration, impaired quality of life, lower respiratory tract infections, aspiration pneumonia, and poor prognosis including prolonged hospital stay and enhanced morbidity and mortality in several phenotypes of older patients ranging from independently living older people, hospitalized older patients and nursing home residents. Enhancing bolus viscosity of fluids greatly improves safety of swallow in all these patients. We believe OD should be recognized as a major geriatric syndrome, and we recommend a policy of systematic and universal screening and assessment of OD among older people to prevent its severe complications.

Copyright © 2012 Nestec Ltd., Vevey/S. Karger AG, Basel

Prevalence

Prevalence of oropharyngeal dysphagia (OD) among the elderly is extremely high. Although sufferers are sometimes unaware of their oropharyngeal dysfunction, OD is a highly prevalent clinical condition which may affect up to 30–40% of the population 65 years old or more. More than 16 million US and up to 30 million European older people will require specific care for dysphagia by this year 2011, and we have proposed the recognition of OD as a geriatric syndrome [1]. Prevalence of OD is higher in older patients with neurodegenerative diseases (up to 80%), or stroke (40%) and is also related to age, frailty (44%) and some common comorbidities in older people, such as muscular, endocrine or psychiatric diseases [2]. We recently studied the real prevalence of OD among independently living older persons, and found the following prevalence: OD, 23.0% (16.6% in the 70–79 years group and 33.0% in the ≥80 years group), impaired efficacy of swallow, 16.8% (9.5% in the 70–79 years group and 28.3% in the ≥80 years group), impaired safety of swallow, 11.4% (6.8% in the 70–79 years group and 18.6% in the ≥80 years group), and oropharyngeal aspiration, 0.74% (0% in the 70–79 years group and 4.4% in the ≥80 years group) [3]. Prevalence of OD among elderly hospitalized patients is much higher, and age >75 years doubles the risk of dysphagia and has a significant impact on morbidity and hospital length of stay [4]. We also found dysphagia affected up to 44% of patients admitted to the acute geriatric unit of our hospital and had a significant impact on prognosis and mortality of patients [5]. Dysphagia also affects more than 50% of older people living in nursing homes, and up to 29% of them were tube fed mainly due to severe aspirations [6]. All these data indicate that OD is a prevalent and serious condition among the main phenotypes of older patients.

The current state of the art of OD management among the elderly aims at: (a) the early identification of patients at risk for dysphagia, (b) the assessment of its pathophysiology and the alterations in the swallow response, and (c) the prevention and treatment of the potential complications of dysphagia such as malnutrition, dehydration and aspiration pneumonia (AP).

Pathophysiology

Videofluoroscopy (VFS) is the gold standard for the study of the mechanisms of dysphagia in the elderly. Main observations during VFS are done in the lateral plane while swallowing 5- to 20-ml boluses of a hydrosoluble contrast of at least three consistencies: liquid, nectar and pudding [7–9]. The aim of the VFS study in these older patients is: (a) to evaluate the safety and efficacy of deglutition, (b) to characterize the alterations of deglutition in terms of videofluoroscopic signs, (c) to help select and assess the effect of treatments, and (d) to make accurate measurements of oropharyngeal swallow response [8, 9]. At our institution,

VFS is performed on every older patient with a positive screening for OD using the VVST [10]. VFS can assess several signs related to the transport function of swallowing, the *efficacy of deglutition*, which is the patient's ability to ingest all the calories and water he or she needs to remain adequately nourished and hydrated, and (b) *safety,* which is the patient's ability to ingest all needed calories and water with no respiratory complications [8–12].

The main VFS signs of efficacy of swallowing in the oral preparatory phase are impaired lip closure allowing bolus spillage in 20% of frail older patients and incapacity to form the bolus, which leads to the bolus spreading throughout the entire oral cavity also in 20% [8, 11]. Major signs of impaired efficacy during the oral stage include apraxia and decreased control and bolus propulsion by the tongue with piecemeal deglutition (multiple swallows per bolus). Many older patients present deglutitional apraxia (difficulty, delay or inability to initiate the oral stage) following a stroke [13]. This symptom is also seen in patients with Alzheimer's, dementia and patients with diminished oral sensitivity. Impaired lingual propulsion in the elderly is caused by tongue sarcopenia [14] and leads to oral or vallecular residue in 40 and 60% of older patients with OD, respectively [11]. The main sign regarding safety during the oral stage is glossopalatal (tongue-soft palate) seal insufficiency, a serious dysfunction that results in the bolus falling into the hypopharynx before the triggering of the oropharyngeal swallow response and while the airway is still open, which causes predeglutitive aspiration [1, 8].

Pharyngeal residue is the main VFS sign of efficacy of the pharyngeal phase. Homogeneous residue in the pharynx is a symptom of weak tongue squeeze and reduced pharyngeal clearance, often observed in frail older patients with neuromuscular diseases. In contrast, unilateral residue is a symptom of unilateral pharyngeal dysfunction, and residue in one pyriform sinus shows a weak unilateral pharyngeal contraction; this is a very common sign in patients with stroke [9]. Postdeglutitive residue is an important VFS sign as aspiration after the pharyngeal swallow is the result of ineffective pharyngeal clearance. The VFS signs of reduced safety of the pharyngeal phase are penetrations and aspirations into the airway. A laryngeal penetration occurs when the bolus enters the laryngeal vestibule and aspiration when liquid traverses the true vocal folds and enters the airway. We observed penetration into the laryngeal vestibule during liquid series in up to 55% of frail older patients and tracheobronchial aspiration in up to 15% [11]. The severity of aspirations and penetrations can be further characterized according to Rosenbek's penetration-aspiration scale and according to whether they are followed by cough or not (silent aspirations) [15]. Mechanisms of aspiration are classified as predeglutitive (before activation of pharyngeal phase), intradeglutitive or postdeglutitive [16, 17]. Through VFS, we found serious swallowing and cough reflex disorders in a group of frail elderly patients as more than half presented penetrations of ingested material into the laryngeal vestibule or aspirations beyond the vocal folds during the

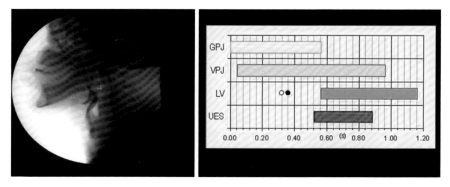

Fig. 1. Representative example of VFS recordings of a 5-ml nectar swallow in a frail older patient with stroke showing an aspiration into the airway as the bolus traverses the vocal cords. Note radiopaque references used to avoid magnification during spatial measurements. Diagram at the right shows temporal events at GPJ, VPJ, LV and UES, defining timing of oropharyngeal swallow response; white dot represents timing of laryngeal penetration and the black dot, time of aspiration.

swallow response, many of which were silent due to simultaneous impairment of cough reflex [11].

From a biomechanical perspective, the two main components of oropharyngeal swallow response are the configuration of the oropharynx from a respiratory to a digestive pathway, and the transfer of the bolus from the mouth to the esophagus which includes bolus propulsion, the opening of the upper esophageal sphincter, and pharyngeal clearance [1]. Quantitative measurements of each one of these components can be easily obtained in the clinical setting with VFS [1, 8, 9, 11, 16]. The normal swallow response is characterized by short duration – less than 1 s –, very fast configuration of the oropharynx from a respiratory to a digestive pathway with early protection of airway and fast laryngeal vestibule closure (LVC) – less than 160 ms –, and strong bolus propulsion by tongue squeeze with high bolus velocity [11]. In contrast, OD in the elderly is mainly characterized by high prevalence of penetrations and aspirations during swallow response, and oropharyngeal residue [11]. Pathophysiology of impaired safety and aspirations is mainly associated with delayed LVC and delayed maximal anterior and vertical hyoid movement (fig. 1), and impaired efficacy is associated with weak tongue squeeze and weak bolus propulsion forces [11]. Future specific treatments for OD in the elderly should be targeted to improve these critical physiological events.

Impaired swallow response in the frail elderly is caused by neurogenic and myogenic factors (table 1). Studies on healthy people over 80 years of age found that normal aging delayed and prolonged swallow response and increased oropharyngeal residue [18–20]. Delayed swallow response has been attributed to impaired function of peripheral afferents to the swallowing center and slow

Clavé · Rofes · Carrión · Ortega · Cabré · Serra-Prat · Arreola

Table 1. Pathophysiology of OD in older persons

	Pathogenesis				Etiology/risk factors
	Function	VFS sign	Physiology	Mechanism	
OD	Impaired safety	• Penetration • Aspiration • Silent aspiration	• Slow GPJO-LVO • Slow LVC • Slow UESO • Slow hyoid motion • Cough reflex	Slow swallow response 'neural'	• Aging • Stroke • Neurodegenerative • Parkinson • Dementia • Confusion • Drugs
	Impaired efficacy	• Lip closure • Tongue control • Tongue propulsion • Piecemeal • Oral residue • Vallecular residue • Pharyngeal residue	• Reduced bolus velocity • Reduced bolus kinetic energy • Reduced bolus size	Weak tongue squeeze 'muscular'	• Sarcopenia • Muscle mass • Frailty • Weakness • Fatigue • Malnutrition • Hypoactivity • Cytokines • Hyper-TGC

synaptic conduction in the central nervous system caused by high prevalence of neurological and neurodegenerative diseases in the elderly as well as the neurodegenerative process related to ageing [21]. Drugs with detrimental effects on consciousness or swallow response can also contribute to delayed swallow response [22]. Weak muscular tongue strength caused by sarcopenia is the major contributor to impaired bolus propulsion [14]. Table 1 summarizes the main elements causing OD in the elderly [1].

Natural History, Prognosis and Complications

OD causes severe and specific complications in several phenotypes of older patients that can lead to death. The impact of OD on the health of older patients is higher than that of other chronic conditions such as metabolic and cardiovascular diseases and even that of some types of cancer [23]. OD may give rise to two groups of clinically relevant complications in older people: (a) malnutrition and/or dehydration caused by a decrease in the efficacy of deglutition, and (b) choking and tracheobronchial aspiration caused by the decrease in deglutition safety and which results in respiratory infections and AP with high mortality rates [1]. Despite this, OD is underestimated and underdiagnosed as a cause of symptoms and major nutritional and respiratory complication in older patients. Figure 2 summarizes the pathophysiology of complications related to dysphagia

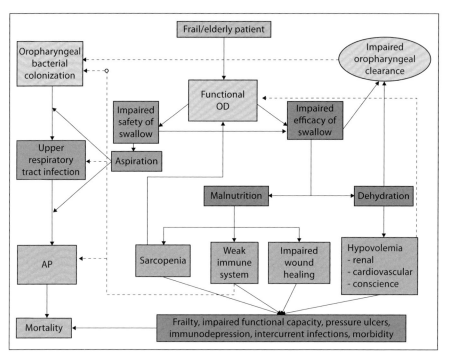

Fig. 2. Nutritional and respiratory complications associated with OD in older patients.

in the elderly [1]. Several studies have evaluated the impact of OD and these specific complications among different phenotypes of elderly people. First, in a transversal study on a cohort of independently living older persons, we found high prevalence of OD was statistically associated with advanced age, low Barthel score, benzodiazepines treatment, depression, slow walking speed, and low overall quality of life (QoL) [3]. Moreover, a close relationship between signs of OD and poor functional capacity was observed and, independent of age and functional capacity, impaired efficacy of swallow was associated with an increased risk of malnutrition [3]. We also performed a longitudinal study with similar patients, and found that prevalence of malnutrition at one-year follow-up was associated with basal OD and with basal signs of impaired efficacy of swallow [24]. Likewise, annual incidence of low respiratory tract infections (LRTIs) was higher in subjects with basal signs of impaired safety of swallow in comparison to subjects without such signs, clearly showing OD is a risk factor for malnutrition and LRTIs in independently living older persons [24]. The social and psychological impact of OD on older patients living in nursing homes in Europe was measured in a study that found a major negative impact of OD on QoL of these patients in that only 45% patients found eating pleasant, 41% felt anxiety or panic during mealtimes, and 36% avoided eating with others because of OD [2].

We also studied the prevalence and clinical impact of OD as a potential geriatric syndrome in 1,160 patients (mean age 84 years) admitted to the geriatric unit of our hospital due to several acute diseases, and found that 44% of older patients presented OD and that the prevalence of malnutrition (33%), weakness, length of stay, impaired functional capacity, morbidity and one-year mortality (40% in patients with OD) was significantly increased in older patients with OD [25]. More recently, in a study using clinical tools, biochemical markers, anthropometric measurements and bioimpedance, we found that 66% of older patients with VFS signs of OD were malnourished or at risk of malnutrition and presented severe depletion of muscular protein and intracellular water showing subclinical dehydration, another very frequent complication in older patients with OD [26].

The impact of OD on prognosis and mortality is especially severe in older patients with AP as one of the consequences. A recent 10-year review found a 93.5% increase in the number of hospitalized older patients diagnosed with AP, while other types of pneumonia in the elderly decreased [27]. AP occurs in the first days following stroke in up to 20% of patients, and is the first cause of one-year mortality after discharge [13, 28]. We studied 134 older patients (>70 years) with pneumonia consecutively admitted to an acute geriatric unit in our general hospital. Of the 134 patients, 53% were >84 years old, and 55% presented clinical signs of OD; the mean Barthel score was 61 points, indicating a frail population. Patients with dysphagia were older, showed lower functional status, higher prevalence of malnutrition and comorbidities, higher Fine's pneumonia severity scores and higher mortality at 30 days (22.9 vs. 8.3%, p = 0.033) and at 1 year of follow-up (55.4 vs. 26.7%, p = 0.001) [22]. OD can thus be considered a highly prevalent clinical finding and an indicator of disease severity in older patients with pneumonia [22]. Also recently, we found VFS signs of impaired safety in up to 54% of older patients admitted to our hospital with community-acquired pneumonia and a marked delay in LVC. In elderly nursing home residents with OD, AP occurs in 43–50% during the first year, with a mortality of up to 45% [28].

Taken together, these results confirm that OD is a major factor for malnutrition, pneumonia, impaired QoL, and other complications including mortality in very different phenotypes of older patients ranging from independently living older subjects to hospitalized patients and older patients living in nursing homes. However, dysphagia with oropharyngeal aspiration is rarely considered a risk factor in elderly patients with community-acquired pneumonia or in elderly patients with malnutrition. We therefore recommend a policy of universal screening for and assessment of OD as part of the standard geriatric evaluation of these patients. We also believe OD fulfills most criteria to be recognized as a major geriatric syndrome as its prevalence is very high in geriatric patients and leads to multiple diseases, risk factors and precipitating diseases, and represents a specific target for therapeutic interventions [29].

Treatment

Identification of videofluoroscopic signs allows the classification of patients with dysphagia into several therapeutic categories ranging from: (a) patients with safe and efficient swallowing that can achieve free oral intake; (b) patients with mild symptoms that need strategies based on the reduction of volume and increase in bolus consistency; (c) patients with severe symptoms that also need changes in head posture, heightened sensory input, and swallow maneuvers, and (d) those patients with such severe aspirations or such inefficient swallowing that they need percutaneous endoscopic gastrostomy in order to avoid respiratory complications or malnutrition [1, 8]. We try to maintain a minimal safe oral intake in these latter patients, with eventual rehabilitation as our aim. The specific indication for each one of these treatments has been summarized recently in a clinical guideline [8]. The strategies for rehabilitation and the effect of therapy by SLP will be discussed in two specific chapters of this volume, and have been recently revised [30]. In the first stage of our research strategy, we assess the therapeutic effect on OD and swallow physiology of the two main therapeutic approaches: (a) changes in bolus volume and viscosity and dietary adjustments [8–11], and (b) new neurophysiologic stimulation treatments based on electrical or pharmacological therapies [1, 31].

We have performed several studies to assess the therapeutic effect of increasing bolus viscosity with thickeners in patients with functional OD. We first calculated the amount of thickener (Resource Thicken Up; Nestlé Healthcare Nutrition, Spain) to be added to the X-ray contrast in order to have appropriate viscosities for the VFS studies: 20.4 mPa•s for liquids, 274.4 mPa•s for nectar, and 3,931.2 mPa•s for pudding [9–11]. We then studied the effect of thickeners on patients with OD caused by non-progressive brain damage (mainly stroke), neuromuscular degenerative diseases including amyotrophic lateral sclerosis, multiple sclerosis or myopathies [9], older patients with neurological, neurodegenerative or head and neck diseases [10], and frail elderly patients [11]. In all these phenotypes of older patients, we found scientific evidence of a strong therapeutic effect on efficacy and safety of oral and pharyngeal phases of swallowing by enhancing bolus viscosity to nectar and a maximal therapeutic effect on safety at pudding viscosity [9–11]. Thickeners minimized the prevalence of VFS signs of impaired safety in frail elderly patients and reduced aspirations from 17% during liquid series to 9% at nectar viscosity and 6% with pudding [11]. In contrast, increasing bolus volume severely impaired safety and efficacy of deglutition, and pudding viscosity increased oropharyngeal residue [11]. Increasing bolus viscosity in these patients did not correct prolonged duration of mechanical components of the oropharyngeal swallow response, and the mechanism of its therapeutic effect seems to be related to an effect of intrinsic bolus characteristics and not to an improvement in the swallow response [9–11]. Taken together, these results show that fluid adaptation should be adopted as a first-line treatment in all older patients with OD, and similar studies should be conducted to demonstrate the potential therapeutic effect of the adaptation of the consistency of solid foods on safety and efficacy of deglutition [1].

In addition, we believe that specific treatments for impaired swallow response in older persons should be developed and assessed. The pathophysiological factors causing dysphagia in the frail elderly can be treated potentially by: (a) the stimulation of TRPV1 receptors located in afferent sensory fibers from the larynx (superior laryngeal nerve) or the pharynx (pharyngeal branch of the glossopharyngeal nerve) by acid, thermal stimulation or specific TRPV1 agonists to speed the neural swallow responses [31]; (b) rehabilitation by lingual resistance exercises, an effective treatment for patients with lingual weakness and dysphagia due to frailty [14], and (c) the classical suprahyoid exercise program (Shaker maneuver) to improve hyoid motion and UES opening [32]. Electrical stimulation of suprahyoid muscles has also improved hyoid and laryngeal elevation [33].

Treatment of dysphagia in older patients varies greatly between centers. This variability can contribute to controversy over the effect of swallowing therapy in preventing malnutrition and AP in older persons. In addition, there are a limited number of studies addressing these – unresolved – questions. We believe that OD in the elderly can be treated, and treatment is cost-effective, and that the use of dysphagia programs is correlated with reduction in the impact of its complications, improvement in nutritional status, reduction in AP rates and mortality, and overall improvement in QoL.

References

1 Rofes L, Arreola V, Almirall J, et al: Diagnosis and management of oropharyngeal dysphagia and Its nutritional and respiratory complications in the elderly. Gastroenterol Res Pract 2011;2011. pii: 818979.

2 Ekberg O, Hamdy S, Woisard V, et al: Social and psychological burden of dysphagia: its impact on diagnosis and treatment. Dysphagia 2002;17:139–146.

3 Serra-Prat M, Hinojosa G, López D, et al: Prevalence of oropharyngeal dysphagia and impaired safety and efficacy of swallow in independently living older persons. J Am Geriatr Soc 2011;59:186–187.

4 Altman KW, Yu GP, Schaefer SD: Consequence of dysphagia in the hospitalized patient: impact on prognosis and hospital resources. Arch Otolaryngol Head Neck Surg 2010;136:784–789.

5 Cabré M, Almirall J, Clavé P: The same patients in various European countries. Aspiration pneumonia: management in Spain. Eur Geriatr Med 2011;2:180–183.

6 Lin LC, Wu SC, Chen HS, et al: Prevalence of impaired swallowing in institutionalized older people in Taiwan. J Am Geriatr Soc 2002;50:1118–1123.

7 Ruiz de León A, Clavé P: Videofluoroscopy and neurogenic dysphagia. Rev Esp Enferm Dig 2007;99:3–6.

8 Clavé P, García Peris P (eds): Guía de diagnóstico y de Tratamiento Nutricional y Rehabilitador de la Disfagia Orofaríngea. Barcelona, Glosa, 2011.

9 Clavé P, de Kraa M, Arreola V, et al: The effect of bolus viscosity on swallowing function in neurogenic dysphagia. Aliment Pharmacol Ther 2006;24:1385–1394.

10 Clavé P, Arreola V, Romea M, et al: Accuracy
of the volume-viscosity swallow test for clinical screening of oropharyngeal dysphagia
and aspiration. Clin Nutr 2008;27:806–815.

11 Rofes L, Arreola V, Romea M, et al:
Pathophysiology of oropharyngeal dysphagia
in the frail elderly. Neurogastroenterol Motil
2010;22:851–858, e230.

12 Logemann JA: Evaluation and Treatment of
Swallowing Disorders, ed 2. Austin, Pro-Ed,
1998.

13 Ickenstein G (ed): Diagnosis and Treatment
of Neurogenic Dysphagia. Uni-Med Verlag,
Bremen, 2011.

14 Robbins J, Langmore S, Hind JA, Erlichman
M: Dysphagia research in the 21st century
and beyond: proceedings from Dysphagia
Experts Meeting, August 21, 2001. J Rehabil
Res Dev 2002;39:543–548.

15 Rosenbek J, Robbins J, Roecker E: A
penetration-aspiration scale. Dysphagia
1996;11:93–98.

16 Kahrilas PJ, Lin S, Rademaker AW,
Logemann JA: Impaired deglutitive airway
protection: a videofluoroscopic analysis of
severity and mechanism. Gastroenterology
1997;113:1457–1464.

17 Medda BK, Kern M, Ren J, et al: Relative
contribution of various airway protective
mechanisms to prevention of aspiration during swallowing. Am J Physiol Gastrointest
Liver Physiol 2003;284:G933–G939.

18 Robbins J, Hamilton JW, Lof GL, Kempster
GB: Oropharyngeal swallowing in normal
adults of different ages. Gastroenterology
1992;103:823–829.

19 Logemann JA, Pauloski BR, Rademaker AW,
et al: Temporal and biomechanical characteristics of oropharyngeal swallow in younger
and older men. J Speech Lang Hear Res
2000;43:1264–1274.

20 Yoshikawa M, Yoshida M, Nagasaki T, et
al: Aspects of swallowing in healthy den-
tate elderly persons older than 80 years.
J Gerontol A Biol Sci Med Sci 2005;60:506–
509.

21 Nagaya M, Sumi Y: Reaction time in the submental muscles of normal older people. J Am
Geriatr Soc 2002;50:975–976.

22 Cabre M, Serra-Prat M, Palomera E, et al:
Prevalence and prognostic implications of
dysphagia in elderly patients with pneumonia. Age Ageing 2010;39:39–45.

23 Goodwin JS, Samet JM, Hunt WC:
Determinants of survival in older cancer
patients. JNCI 1996;88:1031–1038.

24 Serra-Prat AA, Palomera M, Gomez C:
Oropharyngeal dysphagia is a risk factor for
malnutrition and low respiratory tract infec-
tion in independently-living older persons.
A population-based prospective study. Age
Aging 2012;41:376–381.

25 Cabré M, Carrión S, Monteis R, et al:
Prevalence and association between oropharyngeal dysphagia and malnutrition in
patients hospitalized in an acute geriatric
unit (AGU); in Proc 1st Congr ESSD, Leiden,
Sept 2011.

26 Carrión S, Roca M, Areola V, et al:
Nutritional measurements and body composition among patients with oropharyngeal
dysphagia; in Proc 1st Congr ESSD, Leiden,
Sept 2011.

27 Baine WB, Yu W, Summe JP: Epidemiologic
trends in the hospitalization of elderly
Medicare patients for pneumonia, 1991–
1998. Am J Public Health 2001;91:1121–
1123.

28 Cook IJ, Kahrilas PJ: AGA technical review
on management of oropharyngeal dysphagia.
Gastroenterology 1999;116:455–478.

29 Flacker JM: What is a geriatric syndrome
anyway? J Am Geriatr Soc 2003;51:574–576.

30 Speyer R, Baijens L, Heijnen M, Zwijnenberg
I: Effects of therapy in oropharyngeal dysphagia by speech and language therapists: a
systematic review. Dysphagia 2010;25:40–65.

31 Rofes L, Arreola V, Clavé P: Pharmacological
treatment of oropharyngeal dys-
phagia through TRPV1 stimulation.
Neurogastroenterol Motil 2010;22(suppl 1):3.

32 Shaker R, Easterling C, Kern M, et al:
Rehabilitation of swallowing by exercise
in tube-fed patients with pharyngeal dysphagia secondary to abnormal UES opening.
Gastroenterology 2002;122:1314–1321.

33 Burnett TA, Mann EA, Stoklosa JB, Ludlow
CL: Self-triggered functional electrical stimulation during swallowing. J Neurophysiol
2005;94:4011–4018.

Cichero J, Clavé P (eds): Stepping Stones to Living Well with Dysphagia.
Nestlé Nutr Inst Workshop Ser, vol 72, pp 67–76,
Nestec Ltd., Vevey/S. Karger AG., Basel, © 2012

Complications of Oropharyngeal Dysphagia: Aspiration Pneumonia

Jordi Almirall[a] · Mateu Cabré[b] · Pere Clavé[c]

[a]Servei de Cures Intensives, Hospital de Mataró, Universitat Autònoma de Barcelona, CIBER Enfermedades Respiratorias, Instituto de Salud Carlos III, [b]Acute Geriatric Unit, Department of Internal Medicine, Hospital de Mataró, [c]Unitat de Proves Funcionals Digestives, Hospital de Mataró, Universitat Autònoma de Barcelona, CIBER de Enfermedades Hepáticas y Digestivas, Instituto de Salud Carlos III, Barcelona, Spain

Abstract

The incidence and prevalence of aspiration pneumonia (AP) are poorly defined. They increase in direct relation with age and underlying diseases. The pathogenesis of AP presumes the contribution of risk factors that alter swallowing function and predispose to the oropharyngeal bacterial colonization. The microbial etiology of AP involves *Staphylococcus aureus, Haemophilus influenzae* and *Streptococcus pneumoniae* for community-acquired AP and Gram-negative aerobic bacilli in nosocomial pneumonia. It is worth bearing in mind the relative unimportance of anaerobic bacteria in AP. When we choose the empirical antibiotic treatment, we have to consider some pathogens identified in oropharyngeal flora. Empirical treatment with antianaerobics should only be used in certain patients. According to some known risks factors, the prevention of AP should include measures in order to avoid it.

Copyright © 2012 Nestec Ltd., Vevey/S. Karger AG, Basel

Introduction

Definition

We speak of aspiration pneumonia (AP) when we have radiological evidence of pulmonary condensation caused by a large quantity of secretions contaminated by pathogenic bacteria that have passed to the tracheobronchial tree in patients with impaired oropharyngeal or gastroesophageal motility [1]. The location of the radiological sign will depend on the posture of the patient at the time of aspiration. If the patient was upright or semi-recumbent, the affected part will be in the basal segments of the lower lobes, and if the patient was recumbent the most commonly affected areas are in the posterior segment of the upper right lobe and/or the apical segment of the lower right lobe [2].

Incidence and Prevalence of Aspiration Pneumonia
The incidence and prevalence of AP is little known as most epidemiological studies on pneumonia consider cause from aspiration to be criteria for exclusion. In population-based studies, AP accounts for 1.2% of all community-acquired pneumonia (CAP) in persons >14 years of age, an incidence which increases with age [3]. Considering CAP patients who require hospitalization, AP is the cause of 6% of cases, and can reach 10% in patients over 80 years of age [4]. Nursing home residents and particularly those considered frail, however, are most at risk of pneumonia with an incidence of up to 10 times greater than in non-institutionalized older persons [5], with corresponding increased mortality. AP affects more than 30% of patients with stroke and is the main cause of mortality in the first year. About 60–80% of patients with neurodegenerative diseases suffer chronic aspiration of oropharyngeal secretions and the retention of secretions or pneumonia, and AP is the main cause of mortality. It is also the third cause of mortality in patients over 85 years of age [6].

Pathophysiology and Risk Factors

The material aspirated into the tracheobronchial tree must be colonized by bacteria for AP to occur [7]. Aspiration of sterile secretions may cause chemical pneumonitis [4] but not pneumonia. The pathogenesis of AP thus depends on the coexistence of two main groups of risk factors (fig. 1): (a) factors that affect oropharyngeal and/or gastroesophageal motility and (b) factors that favor bacterial colonization in oropharyngeal or gastroesophageal secretions. In the present chapter, we will mainly describe those factors that can influence oropharyngeal colonization.

Risk Factors for Oropharyngeal Colonization
Age
Age increases oropharyngeal colonization by certain bacteria such as *Staphylococcus aureus* and aerobic Gram-negative bacilli (GNB) such as *Klebsiella pneumoniae* and *Escherichia coli* associated with greater comorbidity [8].

Poor Dental Hygiene
The relation between dental and respiratory infection is well known. El-Solh et al. [7] found that there was an 80% coincidence between the bacteria found in the respiratory tract and in the dental plaque of patients from nursing homes who were admitted to the intensive care unit (ICU). ICU patients also had greater risk of nosocomial pneumonia when they had bacterial colonization of

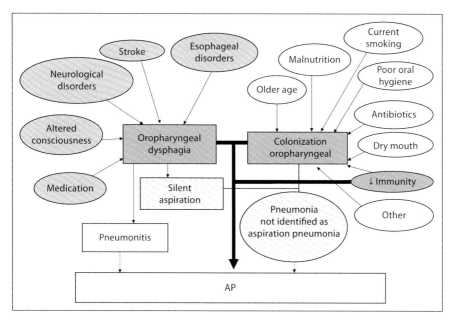

Fig. 1. Known risk factors of AP.

dental plaque [9], and the risk was reduced with prophylactic antiseptic treatment. This suggests that dental plaque which has been colonized by aerobic micro-organisms acts as a microbe reservoir [10], and it follows that it is more evident in patients with dental prostheses than those with their own teeth.

Malnutrition
In addition to being directly related to dysphagia, malnutrition, evaluated from albumin levels and/or body mass index, can be an independent risk factor for pneumonia [11]. Malnutrition has also been described as a factor for poor prognosis associated with a higher mortality rate at 30 days, is clearly associated with mortality at 1 year and very closely associated with the presence of oropharyngeal dysphagia [12]. Thus, dependence, dysphagia, malnutrition and immune status must be considered as major prognostic indicators in elderly patients with pneumonia, as also indicated by other authors [11]. The influence nutrition, particularly vitamin content, has on the immune system could be the cause, although this hypothesis needs to be confirmed in further studies designed to this end.

Smoking
A direct relation, independent of other factors, has been found between smoking and the appearance of CAP [13], and this influence disappears when the habit is given up. The reason for this may be that smoking influences the mechanisms

of the defense system of the host and/or the surface of the mucosa in the respiratory tract by either increasing the number of abnormal cilia or impairing the permeability of the epithelium and thus weakening cilia clearing and favoring bacterial adhesion and consequent colonization.

Antibiotherapy

Several studies on patients diagnosed with CAP have found that antibiotherapy prior to diagnosis affected respiratory infection by some bacteria [14]. This effect was attributed to the selection of oropharyngeal flora with the appearance of more virulent microorganisms.

Inhalers and Aerosols

The devices used to administer treatment to patients with asthma or chronic bronchopathologies can be the source of oropharyngeal contamination as our group recently demonstrated in a case-control study [15]. We found that the role of the inhaled drugs as risk factors for CAP seemed to differ according to the baseline respiratory disease. Inhaled anticholinergics but not inhaled steroids favored CAP in patients with asthma, while inhaled steroids increased the risk for CAP in COPD patients but not in chronic bronchitis patients. This was in agreement with the hypothesis that poor hygiene may represent a causal component of the mechanism of infection. Indeed, the effect of inhalers on the development of CAP can be attributed to the active medication contained in the metered-dose inhaler.

Dehydration

Salivary flow and deglutition play a major role in preserving normal oropharyngeal flora by eliminating GNB. Insufficient liquid intake or decreased salivary production may impair this in older patients with functional incapacity [16] or under certain medication (diuretics, antihistamines, anticholinesterases, antidepressants and drugs for Parkinson's and hypertension), with the consequent increase in bacteria in the oropharyngeal cavity.

Reduction in the Effectiveness of the Immune System

Related to age, the peripheral T cells show signs of weakness when competing with antigens [17].

Special Situations

Nasogastric Tubes. The biofilm on the outer surface favors growth of microorganisms and increases the possibility of septic pseudoembolism in the oropharyngeal cavity, altering the oropharyngeal ecosystem and increasing colonization of the upper airways [18].

Increased Gastric pH. Although gastric juices are sterile due to their acidity, the pH can increase, favoring gastric and oropharyngeal colonization [19].

Almirall · Cabré · Clavé

This has been described in patients with gastroparesis, small-bowel obstruction, enteral nutrition or those under treatment with anti-H_2 or proton pump inhibitors. However, we must be careful when relating acid suppressants, particularly proton pump inhibitors, with pneumonia as the study has been criticized for not using an appropriate control group.

Orotracheal Intubation. The risk of developing nosocomial pneumonia in intubated patients in the ICU is 5 times greater than those not intubated, and is directly related to the duration of intubation [20] and to the need for reintubation. The process can be explained in the following way: bacteria from the pharynx and stomach contaminate subglottic secretions, creating a reservoir which can be aspirated to the trachea, forming a biofilm around the endotracheal tube and which can then be disseminated in the lung through mechanical ventilation.

Microbiology of Aspiration Pneumonia

Basically, the pathogens that contaminate the nasopharynx and oropharynx are those responsible for AP [1]. Strong correlation has been found between cultures of dental plaque samples and those of bronchoalveolar lavage in patients with nosocomial pneumonia associated with mechanical ventilation. The most common are *Haemophilus influenzae* and *Streptococcus pneumoniae*, but in older persons the upper airways can be colonized by aerobic GNB (enterobacteria and *Pseudomonas aeruginosa*) and Gram-positive cocci such as *S. aureus*. Oropharyngeal colonization by aerobic GNB can affect 22–37% of nursing-home residents; the same occurs in patients admitted to the ICU where 60–73% of those over 65 years of age have been found to be contaminated with microorganisms [21]. These groups of patients also have a greater overall risk of infection by resistant *S. pneumoniae*. However, it is difficult to find large series of AP with microbiological diagnosis due to the difficulty of applying invasive fibrobronchoscopial techniques. In two recent studies on AP patients, where the authors used similar methodology [22] with cultures of bronchial secretions obtained with a telescopic catheter, 31 pathogens were isolated from a total of 77 patients. The most diagnosed were *S. aureus*, *H. influenzae* and *S. pneumoniae* in extra hospital pneumonia, and aerobic GNB *(Klebsiella pneumoniae, Escherichia coli, Serratia narcenses* and *Proteus mirabilis)* in nosocomial pneumonia. It is worth noting the scarce implication of anaerobic pathogens contrary to earlier belief [22]. In a recent series by El-Solh et al. [23] on 95 nursing home residents over 65 years of age that were admitted to the ICU for AP, microbiological diagnosis obtained for 54 patients revealed 20% were anaerobic (6 *Prevotella* sp, 3 *Fusobacterium* sp, 1 *Bacteroides* sp and 1 *Peptostreptococcus* s), but the majority also had enteric GNB, and the authors emphasized the clinical resolution within 72 h without the use of anaerobicides. This differs from studies published in the 1970s in which anaerobic pathogens were given greater importance, but the methodology employed then is being questioned now [2]: microbiological cultures were made on samples obtained by transtracheal puncture which only revealed one contamination. They were also performed when the infection was advanced, often following complications such as abscesses, necrotizing pneumonia or empyema and on patients with chronic alcoholism most of whom presented purulent sputum, quite different from the patients we usually treat nowadays.

Antibiotic Treatment of Aspiration Pneumonia
The choice of antibiotic depends on the place of acquisition of AP and the patient's prior state of health. Although AP is often treated empirically with penicillin or clindamycin, this may be inadequate for most AP given the normal microorganisms of the oropharyngeal flora such as *S. pneumoniae, H. influenzae* and GNB. The need for empirical treatment of anaerobic pathogens is not demonstrated as several studies have shown better clinical results without this antibiotic treatment. In any case, this treatment should be reserved for patients with major periodontal disease, purulent sputum or radiological evidence of necrotizing pneumonia or lung abscess. Nevertheless, the current guidelines for the treatment of suspected AP [24] recommend using intravenous amoxicillin-clavulanic acid (2 g amoxicillin/8 h) for 14 days. Moxifloxacin, ertapenem or clindamycin with a third-generation cephalosporin are alternatives. Cephalosporin should be replaced by piperacillin-tazobactam combination if ICU admission is needed. Above all, possible local resistances must be taken into account and treatment adjusted accordingly.

Prevention

Prevention and treatment of AP are currently possible. According to the two pathophysiological pillars on which the appearance of AP is based, we can intervene both in the prevention of oropharyngeal and gastropharyngeal colonization and in the treatment of oropharyngeal dysphagia which allow endobronchial aspiration (fig. 2). We can prevent oropharyngeal colonization in the following ways:

1 Administration of antipneumococcic and anti-influenza vaccines, preferably together.
2 Meal programs can improve nutritional risk and results suggest that such interventions may help reduce risk of CAP in older persons.
3 Advise giving up smoking.
4 Care of oral hygiene has been shown to reduce colonization by virulent pathogens and the incidence of pneumonia. Intensive oral hygiene improves

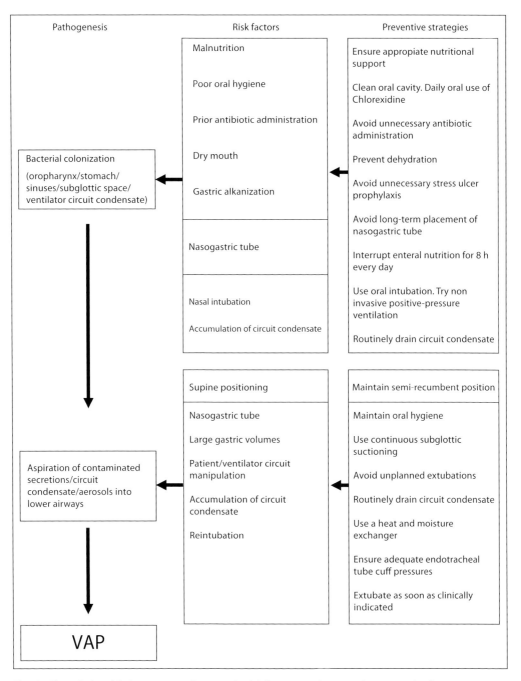

Fig. 2. The relationship between pathogenesis, risk factors, and preventive strategies for ventilator-associated pneumonia (VAP).

sensitivity to cough reflex as the changes produced by contaminating pathogens in the mucous and nerve endings are improved. Programs to clean dental prostheses should be established as well as the habit of wearing dentures during daytime only [25]. Oral hygiene should be maintained even among edentulous patients as 'tongue cleaning' is associated with decreased oropharyngeal bacterial load.

5 Nasogastric tubes do not prevent aspiration in patients with dysphagia and advanced dementia and so should only be used when strictly necessary. With regard to 24-hour enteral nutrition, interruptions of 6 h are recommended so the gastric pH can return to normal and eradicate bacteria that could otherwise cause oropharyngeal contamination [21].

6 Hand washing with antibacterial soap (chlorhexidine) followed by alcoholic solution before and after contact with the patient.

7 Avoid administration of sedatives in order to prevent relaxation of the oropharyngeal musculature. Antihistamines and anticholinergics should also be avoided.

8 Maintenance of good hydration of the oral cavity.

9 Avoid unnecessary antibiotic treatment although there is not enough evidence yet to show a reduction in the incidence of pneumonia.

10 Prophylaxis with anti-H_2 and proton bomb inhibitors should be restricted to patients who present recurrent pneumonia during treatment, at least until more scientific evidence is available [26].

11 Maintenance of good hygiene and dryness of pressurized devices and aerosols used in bronchodilator therapy.

12 Noninvasive mechanical ventilation in patients admitted for respiratory insufficiency is preferable as, among other advantages, it has a lower incidence of nosocomial pneumonia.

13 Subglottic aspirations are effective in patients that require more than 3 days' orotracheal intubation. Selective digestive decontamination (mouth and stomach) with polymyxin + aminoglycoside + amphotericin is recommended to reduce the gastric bacterial load and avoid tracheobronchial colonization, thus reducing the incidence of pneumonia associated with mechanical ventilation. Similar results have been published on the decontamination of the oral cavity with chlorhexidine or chlorhexidine + colistin. Studies that question these results have prevented generalized use, but considering cost/benefits and the fact that they do not induce resistance to antibiotics, oral decontamination with chlorhexidine is an attractive method of reducing pneumonia.

14 Consider raising hospitalized patients in bed to a 45° angle [27], even though effectiveness has not been demonstrated in patients outside the ICU.

References

1   Tuomanen EI, Austrian RR, Masure HR: Pathogenesis of pneumococcal infection. N Engl J Med 1995;332:1280–1284.

2   Marik PE: Aspiration pneumonitis and aspiration pneumonia. N Engl J Med 2001;344:665–6715.

3   Almirall J, Bolibar I, Vidal J, et al: Epidemiology of community-acquired pneumonia in adults: a population-based study. Eur Respir J 2000;15:757–763.

4   Fernandez-Sabé N, Carratalà J, Rosón B, et al: Community-acquired pneumonia in very elderly patients: causative organisms, clinical characteristics, and outcomes. Medicine 2003;82:159–169.

5   Quagliarello V, Ginter S, Han L, et al: Modifiable risk factors for nursing home-acquired pneumonia. Clin Infect Dis 2005;40:1–6.

6   Cabre M, Serra-Prat M, Bolibar I, et al: Prognostic factors of community acquired pneumonia in very old patients. Med Clin (Barc) 2006;127:201–205.

7   El-Solh AA, Pietrantoni C, Bhat A, et al: Colonization of dental plaques. A reservoir of respiratory pathogens for hospital-acquired pneumonia in institutionalized elders. Chest 2004;126:1575–1582.

8   Valenti WM, Trudell RG, Bentley DW: Factors predisposing to oropharyngeal colonization with gram negative bacilli in the aged. N Engl J Med 1978;298:1108–1111.

9   Fourrier F, Duvivier B, Boutigny H, et al: Colonization of dental plaque: a source of nosocomial infections in intensive care unit patients. Crit Care Med 1998;26:301–308.

10 Russell SL, Boylan RJ, Kaslick RS, et al: Respiratory pathogen colonization of the dental plaque of institutionalized elders. Spec Care Dent 1999;3:262–275.

11 Hiramatsu K, Niederman MS: Health care-associated pneumonia: a new therapeutic paradigm. Chest 2005;128:3784–3787.

12 Cabre M, Serra-Prat M, Palomera E, et al: Prevalence and prognostic implications of dysphagia in elderly patients with pneumonia. Age and Ageing 2009;39:39–45.

13 Almirall J, Gonzalez CA, Balanzó X, et al: Proportion of community-acquired pneumonia cases attributable to tobacco smoking. Chest 1999;116:375–379.

14 Almirall J, Bolibar I, Serra-Prat M, et al: New evidence of risk factors for community acquired pneumonia: a population-based study. Eur Respir J 2008;31:1274–1284.

15 Almirall J, Bolíbar I, Serra-Prat M, et al: Inhaled drugs as risk factors for community-acquired pneumonia. Eur Respir J 2010;36:1080–1087.

16 Palmer LB, Albulak K, Fields S, et al: Oral clearance and pathogenic oropharyngeal colonization in the elderly. Am J Respir Crit Care Med 2001;164:464–468.

17 Saltzman RL, Peterson PK: Immunodeficiency of the elderly. Rev Infect Dis 1987;9:1127–1139.

18 Leibovitz A, Plotikov G, Habot B, et al: Pathogenic colonization of oral flora in frail elderly patients fed by nasogastric tube or percutaneous enterogastric tube. J Gerontol A Biol Sci Med Sci 2003;58:52–55.

19 Laheij RJF, Sturkenboom MCJM, Hassing RJ, et al: Risk of community-acquired pneumonia and use of gastric acid-suppressive drugs. JAMA 2004;292:1955–1960.

20 Fleming CA, Balaguera HU, Craven DE: Risk factors for nosocomial pneumonia: focus on prophylaxis. Med Clin North Am 2001;85:1545–1563.

21 Janssens JP, Krause KH: Pneumonia in the very old. Lancet Infect Dis 2004;4:112–124.

22 Marik PE, Careau P: The role of anaerobes in patients with ventilator-associated pneumonia and aspiration pneumonia: a prospective study. Chest 1999;115:178–183.

23 El-Solh A, Pietrantoni C, Bhat A, et al: Microbiology of severe aspiration pneumonia in institutionalized elderly. Am J Respir Crit Care Med 2003;167:1650–1654.

24 Mandell LA, Wunderink RG, Anzueto A, et al: Infectious Diseases Society of America/American Thoracic Society Consensus Guidelines on the Management of Community-Acquired Pneumonia in Adults. Clin Infect Dis 2007;44:S27–S72.

25 Budtz-Jorgensen E, Mojon P, Rentsch A, Deslauriers N: Effects of an oral health program on the occurrence of oral candidosis in a long-term care facility. Community Dent Oral Epidemiol 2000;28:141–149.

26 CAG Clinical Affairs Committee. Community-acquired pneumonia and acid-suppressive drugs: position statement. Can J Gastroenterol 2006;20:119–121.

27 Drakulovic MB, Torres A, Bauer TT, et al: Supine body position as a risk factor for nosocomial pneumonia in mechanically ventilated patients: a randomised trial. Lancet 1999;354:1851–1858.

Cichero J, Clavé P (eds): Stepping Stones to Living Well with Dysphagia.
Nestlé Nutr Inst Workshop Ser, vol 72, pp 77–83,
Nestec Ltd., Vevey/S. Karger AG., Basel, © 2012

Nutrition Assessment and Intervention in the Patient with Dysphagia: Challenges for Quality Improvement

Juan B. Ochoa

Nestlé HealthCare Nutrition, Nestlé Health Science, Florham Park, NJ, USA

Abstract

Dysphagia, a symptom characterized by difficulty swallowing, is an independent predictor of poor outcome, worsening morbidity, increasing the risk for hospital readmissions, health care costs and mortality. Dysphagia is a result of a number of illnesses including neurological diseases, after surgery for head and neck pathology, observed in the intensive care unit after prolonged endotracheal intubation among others, and is particularly frequent in the elderly. Dysphagia increases the incidence of malnutrition, which in turn delays patient recovery. Treatment of dysphagia can be successful, but requires the use of multidisciplinary teams. A focus on the management of malnutrition including prevention and treatment is essential. Perhaps the biggest challenge is the lack of awareness of the presence of dysphagia and malnutrition, so that only a minority of patients are identified and successfully treated. We propose that better identification and treatment of dysphagia could occur with the systematic implementation of clinical practice improvement processes with a consequent decrease in morbidity, mortality and cost.

Copyright © 2012 Nestec Ltd., Vevey/S. Karger AG, Basel

Introduction

Dysphagia is a prominent symptom associated with multiple illnesses. Neurological conditions, including stroke, account for a large number of cases. However, multiple illnesses including head and neck cancer and prolonged intubation in the intensive care unit also add up significant numbers of patients. Dysphagia can occur at all ages, though in our hospitals and institutions, it is a prominent symptom in the elderly.

The symptom of dysphagia is an independent predictor of poor prognosis. As described by Altman [this volume, pp. 119–126], patients with dysphagia exhibit increased length of stay in the hospitals, increased complication rates and utilization of resources, and more frequently require institutionalized care. The utilization of health care resources including nursing homes and rehabilitation facilities is significantly increased in patients with dysphagia. There is a consequent increase in cost, which is difficult to define but may constitute hundreds of millions of dollars in the USA alone [1].

Although dysphagia is only a symptom, the biological consequences that arise from this are significant. Dysphagia is associated with aspiration and the development of pneumonia, an illness that may require hospitalization and be the cause of death in these patients. Patients with dysphagia become socially isolated contributing to the emergence of symptoms of depression [2].

Malnutrition and Dysphagia

The lack of adequate nutrition is prominent in patients with dysphagia. An evaluation of 8 different trials reported by Foley et al. [3] in stroke patients for example, demonstrated that patients with dysphagia were 2.4 times more likely to develop malnutrition, which became clinically prominent during rehabilitation and recovery. These data suggest that patients with onset of dysphagia are at significant risk of progressing towards malnutrition.

Malnutrition contributes to worsening prognosis in all illnesses, and patients with dysphagia are no exception. Malnutrition worsens the immune system's capacity to heal, negatively affects muscle function (particularly respiratory efforts) and delays or prevents adequate recovery [4]. Pneumonia is a complication of dysphagia and significantly worsened in patients with malnutrition.

Malnutrition in patients with dysphagia possibly occurs as a result of several mechanisms. Traditional belief dictates that malnutrition occurs as a result of poor oral intake and is the result of prolonged starvation. This, starvation-related malnutrition is traditionally observed in the third world due to lack of availability of nutrients and caused by natural disasters or political strife. In developed countries, starvation-related malnutrition is not frequently acknowledged, and thus may not be adequately diagnosed. Starvation-related malnutrition occurs in patients with dysphagia who will be incapable of eating as a result of impairment in maintaining activities of daily living such as that seen in patients with neurological diseases. It can also be the result of progressive aversion to eating as the result of choking and pulmonary impairment.

Starvation-related malnutrition is treated with adequate food replacement. Every effort should be done at adequate prevention. Physicians appropriately focus on patient stabilization and treatment of the acute illness (after a stroke for example). As a result, the provision of adequate nutrition is of secondary importance. Common clinical practices suppress oral intake maintaining the patient nil per os for days or sometimes even longer. As a result, a caloric deficit rapidly accumulates. Work performed by Villet, and observations by other investigators demonstrate that accumulation of a caloric deficit portends poor prognosis. In addition, policies aimed at providing early oral or enteral nutrient intake are associated with improved outcomes including decreased mortality and cost. Ideally, a plan for provision of adequate nutrition should be instituted within the first 12 h of arrival of the patient to the hospital, through execution of protocols and dedicated personnel [5].

For many years, it has been clear that inflammation (either acute or chronic) is a significant cause of malnutrition. Disease-related malnutrition is observed in multiple illnesses, and is the result of immune activation, changes in the hormonal milieu and alterations of the central and autonomic nervous systems. These acute responses have only been partially studied, but are characterized by hyperglycemia and insulin resistance, increased metabolic activity and an increase in muscle destruction and utilization of amino acids to generate glucose (gluconeogenesis). Inflammatory responses hasten the progression towards malnutrition [6].

Attempts at curtailing inflammation-related malnutrition were initially focused on providing larger amounts of energy beyond normal required caloric goals, mostly in the form of glucose and lipids. To support these attempts, nutrition intervention strategies included the use of 'hyperalimentation' through both parenteral and enteral routes. There is no evidence however, that strategies aimed at provision of large amounts of energy above normal needs curtails the catabolic response, or is of any physiological benefit. On the contrary, with few exceptions (such as seen in burns) the practice of providing large amounts of energy is associated with worsening of outcomes and should be abandoned.

The best treatment available at preventing inflammation-related malnutrition is that of controlling the inflammatory response. This is best done by adequately managing the disease and the prevention of subsequent complications such as infections. Limiting the amount of tissue damage during surgery, resecting necrotic tissues, draining abscesses and adequate pain control with the use of multimodality therapy are central to the prevention of disease-related malnutrition. Attempts at controlling the neurohormonal responses are difficult, but have met with some limited success under strict circumstances. Such is the case of the use of beta adrenergic blockade in burn patients.

Advances in nutritional sciences have led to the identification that certain nutrients exhibit 'pharmacologic' properties and modulate immune responses. Immunonutrition, as this specialized area of nutrition intervention is called, offers exciting and important possibilities. Some nutrients that are currently being utilized include amino acids such as arginine and glutamine, certain lipids such as omega-3 fatty acids, micronutrients such as vitamin C and nucleotides. The use of these different nutrients is beyond the scope of this article and the reader is urged to consult other texts [7].

Nutrition Intervention in Dysphagia: A Quality Practice Improvement Process

The application of the scientific method in medicine has used two traditional approaches to successfully develop new treatments. The first uses basic sciences aimed at testing mechanistic hypotheses (i.e. how it works); the second uses clinical research aimed at determining the effectiveness of a specific treatment (i.e. whether it works). Clinical research generates the evidence of clinically relevant benefit through the performance of randomized trials, which are often summarized through meta-analyses. The use of these 'evidence-based' treatments is in turn encouraged through the creation of guidelines protocols and recommendations, many of them supported by professional organizations [8].

The fact that a specific treatment generates clinical benefit, however, does not guarantee widespread adoption by clinicians. In fact, a highly significant concern for all is the realization that adoption of new high-quality knowledge into daily clinical practice may be frustratingly slow. As a result, the benefits of modern medicine may fail to reach many patients. Examples of this abound. Hand washing is only routinely used by a proportion of physicians despite the fact that it evidently decreases nosocomial infections. Elevating the head of the bed in critically ill patients improves outcomes, though again and again practices and institutions fail to adopt these practices. In addition to the obvious negative effects on outcome, failing to improve the quality of care through adoption of scientifically proven effective therapies imposes dramatic increases in cost, which are intolerable in an already taxed health care system [9].

Quality practice improvement is the name given to the discipline aimed at hastening the adoption of effective therapies into daily clinical use. Quality practice improvement draws knowledge from many areas including engineering, social sciences, psychology and others. Industry has for many years understood the importance of quality control and the adoption of careful monitoring of assembly processes. The airline industry has established rigorous quality processes to create a safe mode of transportation. Recently, the government, third party payers and professional organizations have embraced quality practice improvement as a method to reduce medical errors, improve outcomes and decrease cost (http://www.ahrq.gov/).

The management of dysphagia requires careful coordination of multidisciplinary teams, rigorous adherence to protocols and support by institutions, and recognition of their cost-effectiveness by third party payers and government. Adequate nutrition intervention is essential for outcome improvement; as explained above, however, it is difficult for a primary health care team to provide for this care. Quality practice improvement in nutrition could help solve the complexity of nutrition delivery to the bedside in patients with dysphagia.

Nutrition intervention in dysphagia requires a long-term continuum of care. Multiple nutrition-related decisions have to be made during the hospitalization

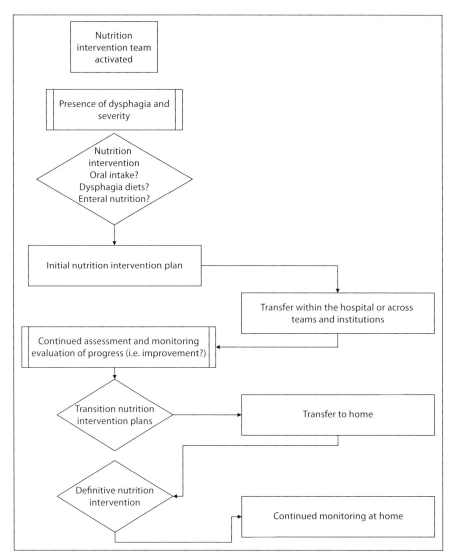

Fig. 1. An example of a flow chart for continued nutrition assessment and intervention of the patient with dysphagia.

and recovery of the patient and eventual return to an independent living. Take the stroke patient, for example. Acute interventions demand airway protection, endotracheal intubation and ventilation if necessary, hemodynamic stabilization, and complex procedures such as angiograms and placement of intravascular stents. During traditional patient care, nutrition intervention is discussed and adopted by the primary team. A decision to allow oral nutrition intake or place a feeding tube has to be made by the primary team [10]. Consultation to a speech pathologist who is not part of the primary team may be required and a decision to initiate nutrition intervention is often delayed until the capacity to swallow is assessed by the consulting service. Nutrition intervention is then started and monitored by the intensive care service. A new primary team receives the patient to a regular floor once he/she leaves the intensive care unit. Nutrition requirements will change for this patient, and decisions of route of intake (oral, enteral, parenteral) will be required. Interventions such as the need for placement of gastrostomies for the provision of long-term enteral nutrition need to be made. The next step in this theoretical patient's journey may require the admission to a skilled nursing facility or to a rehabilitation service where once again, a different nutrition intervention plan will need to be designed and instituted. Finally, the patient will hopefully be able to return home. At home, adequate provision of nutrition will be expected from the patient or his/her family. For example, will the patient require modification of the consistency of liquids and meals? Who and how is hydration going to be monitored? Is the patient taking in enough calories?

The exercise above demonstrates the complexity of providing adequate nutrition assessment and intervention in a patient with dysphagia is quite complex with multiple 'intervention points' and a complex 'flow' of information. Multiple delays and errors in intervention can occur. Quality improvement can significantly improve the quality of intervention and avoid errors. Quality improvement would dictate that a nutrition intervention team would be in charge of all the nutrition-related care of the patient once notified by the primary team upon arrival of the patient. The use of a nutrition team allows for measuring compliance with early nutrition assessments and intervention, seamless transitions through hospitalization, rehabilitation and return to home, detection of any nutrition-related complications and monitoring the cost of nutrition-related health care.

Quality practice improvement has shown significant benefits for the patients and decreased cost for the health care system. Infection rates have significantly decreased in intensive care units that systematically use sterile procedures and careful antibiotic management under the supervision of an infection prevention team. Improved outcomes are observed in surgical practices, showing decreased needs for reintervention and readmissions. Quality practice improvement in nutrition should lead to further improvement in the care of the dysphagia patient [10].

Conclusions

Dysphagia is a poorly recognized symptom that affects multiple patient populations and increases health care costs. Among the negative consequences of dysphagia is the progression towards malnutrition, which in turn worsens prognosis. Nutrition assessment and intervention should be started early and continued throughout the care of the patient and his/her progression towards independence. Early identification of dysphagia should lead to the design of the most appropriate nutrition intervention regimens for the patient and the prevention of progression towards malnutrition increasing the patient's chances for an uneventful recovery and decreasing health care costs.

References

1 Altman KW: Dysphagia evaluation and care in the hospital setting: the need for protocolization. Otolaryngol Head Neck Surg 2011;145:895–898.

2 Cabre M, Serra-Prat M, Palomera E, et al: Prevalence and prognostic implications of dysphagia in elderly patients with pneumonia. Age Ageing 2010;39:39–45.

3 Foley NC, Martin RE, Salter KL, Teasell RW: A review of the relationship between dysphagia and malnutrition following stroke. J Rehabil Med 2009;41:707–713.

4 Rofes L, Arreola V, Almirall J, et al: Diagnosis and management of oropharyngeal dysphagia and its nutritional and respiratory complications in the elderly. Gastroenterol Res Pract 2011;2011. pii: 818979.

5 Villet S, Chiolero RL, Bollmann MD, et al: Negative impact of hypocaloric feeding and energy balance on clinical outcome in ICU patients. Clin Nutr 2005;24:502–509.

6 Jensen GL, Mirtallo J, Compher C, et al: Adult starvation and disease-related malnutrition: a proposal for etiology-based diagnosis in the clinical practice setting from the International Consensus Guideline Committee. JPEN J Parenter Enteral Nutr 2010;34:156–159.

7 Ochoa JB, Makarenkova V, Bansal V: A rational use of immune enhancing diets: when should we use dietary arginine supplementation? Nutr Clin Pract 2004;19:216–225.

8 Horn SD, Gassaway J: Practice-based evidence study design for comparative effectiveness research. Med Care 2007;45(suppl 2):S50–S57.

9 Perry L, McLaren S: Nutritional support in acute stroke: the impact of evidence-based guidelines. Clin Nutr 2003;22:283–293.

10 Miceli BV: Nursing unit meal management maintenance program. Continuation of safe-swallowing and feeding beyond skilled therapeutic intervention. J Gerontol Nurs 1999;25:22–36.

Cichero J, Clavé P (eds): Stepping Stones to Living Well with Dysphagia.
Nestlé Nutr Inst Workshop Ser, vol 72, pp 85–99,
Nestec Ltd., Vevey/S. Karger AG., Basel, © 2012

Therapeutic Approach to Malnutrition and Sarcopenia

Rosa Burgos Peláez

Nutritional Support Unit, Hospital Universitari Vall d'Hebron, Barcelona, Spain

Abstract

Sarcopenia is a syndrome characterized by the progressive loss of muscle mass and strength with a risk of undesirable effects such as physical disability, poor quality of life and death, and it is a major contributing factor of disability and loss of independence in the elderly. Its etiopathogenics include different mechanisms that are both intrinsic to the muscle itself and related to changes in the central nervous system, as well as hormonal and lifestyle factors. Several hormones and cytokines affect muscle function and mass. The reduction in testosterone and estrogens associated with ageing speeds up the loss of muscle mass. Growth hormone is also involved in the loss of lean body mass. Although sarcopenia does not completely revert with exercise, the absence of physical activity accelerates muscle mass loss. Diagnosing sarcopenia is hindered by a lack of reliable methods for measuring muscle mass. Different strategies have been tested for its treatment: testosterone replacement therapy/other anabolic androgens, estrogens in women, growth hormone, nutritional treatment and exercise. Of all the therapeutic options available, only resistance training with or without nutritional supplementation has shown its efficacy in increasing skeletal muscle mass.

Copyright © 2012 Nestec Ltd., Vevey/S. Karger AG, Basel

Introduction

Malnutrition is a state of nutrition in which a deficiency, excess (or imbalance) of energy, protein, and other nutrients causes measurable adverse effects on tissue and body form (body shape, size and composition), body function and clinical outcome [1].

Sarcopenia (from the Greek *sarx*, flesh, and *penia*, poverty) is a syndrome characterized by progressive and generalized loss of skeletal muscle mass and strength with a risk of adverse outcomes such as physical disability, poor quality

Table 1. Criteria for the diagnosis of sarcopenia [2]

Diagnosis of sarcopenia
1   Low muscle mass
2   Low muscle strength
3   Low physical performance

Diagnosis is based on documentation of criterion 1 plus criterion 2 or criterion 3

Table 2. Age-related anatomical changes in muscle in the elderly

1   Reduced muscle mass
2   Infiltration by fat and connective tissue
3   Reduced size of type II fibers, with no changes in type I
4   Reduced number of type II fibers
5   Reduced capillary/fiber ratio
6   Accumulation of internal nuclei, ring and split fibers
7   Myofilament and Z line breakdown
8   Sarcoplasmic reticulum and t-tubule system proliferation
9   Accumulation of lipofuscin and rod-shaped structures
10 Reduced number of motor units

of life and death. The European Working Group on Sarcopenia in the Elderly recently defined the diagnostic criteria (table 1) [2].

Note that the two definitions (malnutrition and sarcopenia) do not include low weight, and both can coexist with obesity.

Muscle mass is reduced by approximately 3–8% per decade starting at the age of 30 [3], and this process speeds up from the age of 60 on. This causes the reduced muscle strength and function involved in disability among the elderly. Sarcopenia increases the risk of falls and fractures and susceptibility to injuries, and can thus be the cause of functional dependence and disability in the elderly population. Sarcopenia is a component of frailty syndrome, and one of the leading risk factors for disability and death among the elderly population. Moreover, the reduction in muscle mass is accompanied by other changes in body composition, such as a progressive increase in fatty mass (table 2). These changes have been associated with greater insulin resistance in the elderly, which is involved in the etiopathogenics of type 2 diabetes mellitus, obesity, hyperlipidemia and hypertension in the genetically susceptible population.

Malnutrition and sarcopenia are interrelated in the cycle of frailty. The loss of muscle mass is often a consequence of senescent musculoskeletal changes

Table 3. Measurements of muscle mass, strength, and function in research and practice [2]

Variable	Research	Clinical practice
Muscle mass	Computed tomography Magnetic resonance imaging Dual energy X-ray absorptiometry (DXA) Bioimpedance analysis (BIA) Total or partial body potassium per fat-free soft tissue	BIA DXA Anthropometry
Muscle strength	Handgrip strength Knee flexion/extension Peak expiratory flow	Handgrip strength
Physical performance	Short Physical Performance Battery (SPPB) Usual gait speed Timed get-up-and-go test Stair climb power test	SPPB Usual gait speed Get-up-and-go test

that occur with ageing, and is worsened by diseases and enhanced by weight loss.

Sarcopenia involves a reduction in muscular strength, rest and total energy expenditure. Because of the anorexia that accompanies ageing, chronic malnutrition develops, thereby worsening sarcopenia.

One of the most important difficulties involved in detecting and monitoring sarcopenia is that there is, as yet, no gold standard examination for its measurement. Different diagnostic methods are used in both clinical and investigational settings (table 3), but the diagnostic values of sarcopenia are not clearly established. The Working Group on Sarcopenia in Older People has suggested using normal values obtained in healthy young adults and establishing the cutoff point for the diagnosis of sarcopenia at two standard deviations below the mean reference value.

Several factors affecting the muscle changes associated with ageing have been identified in the development of sarcopenia. On the one hand, genetic factors, albeit not well identified, are involved. On the other, the sexual steroid deficit that occurs with ageing has a major impact on both muscle and bone trophism [4]. The decrease in sex hormones is accompanied by activation of inflammatory mediators that can act as catabolic cytokines for muscle. Growth hormone deficit is also directly involved in the etiopathogenics of sarcopenia, in synergy with the increase in inflammatory mediators and gonad hormone deficit. IGF-I concentrations in the elderly inversely predict the presence of sarcopenia, acting as a protective factor in men. Weight loss exacerbates sarcopenia, causing a greater loss of lean mass in comparison to fatty mass. Moreover, the lost weight recovered by patients usually comprises a greater proportion of fat [5]. However, even with no weight changes, longitudinal studies show progressive loss of muscle mass with ageing [6]. Exercise is inversely and independently related to free fatty mass, especially in women [6]. However, the relationship between spontaneous exercise and muscle mass is further complicated by additional factors such as bodyweight, excess weight and attitude towards exercise.

Different strategies have been tested in the therapeutic approach to sarcopenia [7–9], they include:
1 Replacement therapy with testosterone/other anabolic agents
2 Estrogen replacement therapy
3 Human growth hormone (HGH) replacement therapy
4 Resistance training
5 Nutritional treatment
6 Interventions on cytokines and immune function

Replacement Therapy with Testosterone/Other Anabolic Agents

Testosterone
Low testosterone concentrations are associated with lower fat-free mass, lower appendicular skeletal muscle mass and decreased knee extension strength in hypogonadal males when compared with healthy controls. These findings have been used to justify testosterone replacement treatment in hypogonadal males. Testosterone concentrations progressively decrease with age in the elderly, while SHBG levels increase, thus further decreasing bioavailable testosterone. The prevalence of hypogonadism is 20% in men over 60, and can be as high as 50% in men over 80.

In young hypogonadal males, testosterone replacement therapy is associated with increased lean mass, reduced fatty mass, and increased muscle strength and muscle protein synthesis [10]. However, there is some controversy concerning the ergogenic effect of testosterone therapy in eugonadal males, and changes in body composition have not always been followed by increased muscle strength. Furthermore, some studies using supraphysiological doses of testosterone in hypogonadal patients have obtained results similar to those obtained with resistance exercise.

In the elderly, however, there are doubts concerning the safety of testosterone therapy, especially with regard to the risk to the prostate and cardiovascular diseases. The elderly are more vulnerable to the undesirable effects of testosterone replacement therapy. Testosterone can induce and exacerbate sleep apnea, increase erythrocyte mass, and cause transient fluid retention and gynecomastia. Testosterone can also increase the size of both benign and malignant prostate tumors, and its effect on prostate carcinogenesis is unclear. It is also unclear whether replacement therapy in hypogonadal patients increases cardiovascular risk through its effect on lipid metabolism. Table 4 summarizes some of the main randomized, controlled studies that have used testosterone therapy in males aged >65 years. Most of them were conducted in hypogonadal males, and the results show some increases in lean mass and decreases in fatty mass, but these results are not always accompanied by functional benefits. In the only

Table 4. Testosterone effect on body composition parameters and muscle strength in males

Study	Study type	Age years	Status	Dose of testosterone	Duration	Effects observed
Brill, 2002	RCT, double blinded	68	Hypogonadal	5 mg/day	4 weeks	→ strength → fat mass → sexual function
Kenny, 2000	RCT, double blinded	76	Hypogonadal	5 mg/day TTS	12 months	→ strength ↓ underlying loss of BMD
Clague, 1999	RCT, double blinded	68	Hypogonadal community	200 mg IM/ 2 weeks	12 weeks	→ hand grip strength → leg strength
Snyder, 1999	RCT, double blinded	65	Hypogonadal/ eugonadal	6 mg/day	36 months	1.9 kg ↑ lean mass → leg strength ↑ lumbar but not hip BMD in hypogonadal group only
Sih, 1997	RCT, double blinded	68	Hypogonadal community	200 mg IM/2 weeks	12 months	10% ↑ hand grip strength
Wittert, 2003	RCT, double blinded	69	Hypogonadal community	80 mg/12 h oral	12 months	2% ↑ lean mass ↓ fat mass → grip and leg strength

RCT = Randomized controlled clinical trial; → = remains unchanged; ↑ = increases; ↓ = decreases.

study that included eugonadal patients, the benefits of the treatment on bone mass were found only in the group of patients with hypogonadism. The testosterone was administered intramuscularly by depot injection, transdermally or using a derivative suitable for oral administration (testosterone undecanoate).

The studies that showed an increase in muscle strength after testosterone replacement therapy presented methodological problems such as a lack of a control group, the use of fixed-dose hormones without titrating to maintain normal levels of circulating testosterone, or the involvement of only very small number of patients, thereby not minimizing erroneous results arising from patient learning and/or exercise training problems.

Dehydroepiandrosterone
Dehydroepiandrosterone (DHEA) supplementation is being researched as sarcopenia treatment. DHEA is produced in the adrenal cortex and is a precursor of different sexual steroids. DHEA concentrations progressively decrease after the age of 30 years, giving rise to different studies using DHEA supplementation to revert the pathophysiological changes associated to age. It has been suggested

that DHEA can increase muscle strength by increasing the circulating testosterone/cortisol ratio.

DHEA treatment has been tested in two studies. In the first, 100 mg of DHEA was administered for 6 months to people aged 50–65, obtaining an increase in lean mass and decrease in fatty mass. However, a moderate increase in muscle strength was found only in men, not in women, while testosterone concentrations increased considerably in the latter. The second [11], a randomized and placebo-controlled study, involved administering 50 mg/day of DHEA for one year to both men and women aged 60–80 years. The group did not achieve the results of the previous study, and no increase was found in lean mass based on the measurement of the body's potassium content.

Oxandrolone

Oxandrolone is an androgenic steroid with a powerful anabolic effect that is suitable for oral use. Its main advantage is that it is less hepatotoxic than other oral androgens and it is resistant to hepatic metabolism. Its undesirable effects are mild and transient and include minor increases in transaminases and reduced HDL cholesterol levels.

There are no clinical studies with oxandrolone in elderly patients with sarcopenia, although there are numerous accounts on wasting conditions such as wasting syndrome associated with HIV infection, neuromuscular and other chronic diseases that involve loss of muscle mass. They show that oxandrolone increases protein synthesis in skeletal muscle, muscle function and exercise levels, protein and energy intake and reduces visceral and total fatty mass while improving nitrogen retention. Oxandrolone could therefore be a therapeutic strategy for the treatment of sarcopenia in the elderly.

Androstenedione

Androstenedione is an androgen produced by the adrenal glands and gonads in both men and women. It is synthesized from DHEA and converted into testosterone or estrone. The anticipated results are mediated by an increase in circulating testosterone, so it has been used considerably as an anabolic agent in athletes. No controlled studies have used androstenedione in the elderly, and the few studies published were conducted in young people. The results regarding its efficacy in increasing plasma testosterone levels have been inconsistent, and an increase in protein synthesis or muscle strength has not been found when comparing resistance training with or without androstenedione [12].

Estrogen Replacement Therapy

The prevalence of osteopenia and osteoporosis in women over 50 years is 42 and 17%, respectively. Menopause is associated with a reduction in lean mass and bone mineral density, both of which are related to estrogen deficit. However, there is some controversy concerning the precise role of estrogens in the loss of bone mass, and it is not very clear whether estrogen replacement therapy can prevent or revert such a loss. Moreover, different studies have shown a significant relationship between lean mass and bone mineral density, and women with osteoporosis have less appendicular skeletal muscle mass than controls without osteoporosis. Walsh and colleagues recently showed that sarcopenia is more prevalent in women with osteopenia (25%) and osteoporosis (50%) than in women with normal mineral bone density (0.8%). Women with osteoporosis and sarcopenia are at high risk of disability and fractures, and therapeutic and preventive measures should thus be taken.

Several studies have assessed the effect of estrogen replacement therapy on muscle mass in postmenopausal women. Low doses of estradiol (0.25 mg) have not altered appendicular skeletal muscle mass after 6 months of treatment, and physical activity remained unchanged in a large group of women over 65 years of age [13].

In younger women (mean 55 years), full doses of estrogen/progestagen replacement therapy have been shown to be effective in increasing lean mass and reducing fatty mass after 6 months of treatment. In women receiving long-term estrogen replacement therapy, however, there were no significant differences with regard to lean mass between treated women and untreated controls.

Human Growth Hormone Replacement Therapy

HGH replacement therapy increases muscle mass and strength in young adults with hypopituitarism [14]. In middle-aged people, HGH has an anabolic effect as in adults over 50 years with adult-onset HGH deficit the treatment increases muscle strength in both men and women [15]. As HGH is required for maintaining muscle and bone, and since the elderly population is HGH deficient, it has been suggested that HGH therapy could be useful for treating sarcopenia. Table 5 summarizes some of the studies conducted with HGH in the elderly.

In summary, HGH therapy does not increase muscle mass or strength in elderly patients. Biological improvements (increased lean mass, reduced fatty mass) are achieved, but they are not accompanied by enhanced strength or activities of daily living capabilities. Studies have been conducted combining exercise and HGH administration. Addition of the growth hormone has not been shown to increase the beneficial effect of exercise.

Combined HGH and testosterone therapy has been shown to have a positive impact on muscle mass. The results for muscle strength, however, are not consistent and only small increases were obtained.

Other strategies have been tested to reproduce the effects of the natural pulsatile secretion of HGH, such as the nocturnal pulsatile administration of GHRH. Vittone and colleagues tested intramuscular nocturnal administration

Table 5. Effects of HGH supplementation in elderly subjects

Study	Patients	Treatment	Changes in body composition	Changes in muscle function
Rudman	Healthy 61–81 IGF-I <350 U/l	HGH 0.03 mg/kg 3 days per week for 3 months	↑ HGH 0.03 mg/kg 3 days per week for 3 months ↑8.8% lean mass ↓14.4% fatty mass ↑1.6% bone mass	
Papadakis	Healthy 70–85 IGF-I low	HGH 0.03 mg/kg 3 days per week for 3 months	↑4.4% lean mass ↓12.8% fatty mass	No changes
Taaffe	Healthy 65–82 IGF-I mean 106 +14 weeks Prior exercise	rHGH 0.02 mg/kg for 10 weeks + resistance exercises	No weight changes ↑ lean mass ↓ fatty mass	No changes
Jorgensen	Adult GH deficit	HGH 17 µg/kg for 3 years	↑ weight 8.4 kg	↑ Quadriceps muscle strength
Thompson	Obese post-menopausal women	rHGH 0.025 mg/kg or IGF-I 0.015 mg/kg/0.6 mg/kg	Greater weight and fatty mass loss with GH and high doses of IGF-I ↑ lean mass	

↑ = Increases; ↓ = decreases.

of GHRH for 6 weeks in people aged 64–76 years with low levels of circulating IGF-I. The GH values measured through integrated 12-hour secretion doubled but, surprisingly, circulating IGF-I remained unaltered. The outcome was only a moderate increase in muscle strength in some exercises. Note that there were no significant undesirable effects.

Khorram conducted a randomized, placebo-controlled study to evaluate nocturnal GHRH administration for 5 months in people with a mean age of 66. The results showed an increase in nitrogen balance in both men and women and a modest increase in muscle mass and strength in men. The only striking undesirable effect was transient hyperlipidemia, which reverted when the study ended.

Treatment with IGF-I combined with IGFBP3 has been shown to be useful in a small group of patients as it increases muscle mass and preserves bone mass. The IGF-I/IGFBP3 combination enables the administration of higher doses of IGF-I without causing hypoglycemia. In general, it is a well-tolerated treatment. IGF-I therapy, however, has not been found to be better than HGH treatment in obese elderly women, in whom fat-free mass increased at the expense of numerous undesirable effects.

The undesirable effects of HGH are greater in the elderly:
– Carpal tunnel syndrome
– Gynecomastia
– Hyperglycemia. The diabetogenic effects of HGH are greater in elderly patients, in whom its administration for one week triples insulin secretion during the glucose overload
– Fluid retention; edemas in the lower extremities
– Arthralgia
– Orthostatic hypotension
– High rate of withdrawal from treatment (43% in some studies)

Resistance Training

Resistance strength training in the elderly [16]:
– Increases muscle mass
– Increases muscle strength
– Improves balance
– Improves resistance

Resistance training is a more effective method to increase muscle strength and mass than endurance training. In a crossover study including elderly males with different types of training, it was found that resistance exercise (weight lifting) maintained muscle mass and strength more than other types of exercise (swimming). Compared with young people, resistance training in the elderly increases muscle strength less in absolute terms but to a similar extent in relative terms. High-intensity exercises (70–80% of maximum capacity) have been found to be the most effective [17]. The mean time to achieving positive effects is 10–12 weeks, although some studies have found it to be after 2 weeks of training. Some physicians are reluctant to recommend this type of exercise to the elderly, but it has been shown that, with appropriate training, they are completely safe even for the very old [18]. Few undesirable effects have been reported, and such exercise would only have to be limited in patients with congestive heart failure.

Table 6 summarizes the main studies that have used resistance training to evaluate its effect on muscle strength in the elderly.

Exercise must be accompanied by sufficient protein intake [19, 20]. The elderly population often consumes less protein than the recommended daily intake for adults (0.8 g protein/kg of weight per day). Elderly people also have a higher protein catabolism rate, and their protein requirements are likely to be higher than those of the non-elderly adult population. Some studies have shown a synergic effect between protein supplementation and physical exercise [18], and insufficient protein intake has probably prevented better exercise outcomes.

Table 6. Effects of resistance training on muscle strength in elderly subjects

Study	Type of study	Gender	Mean age	Type of training	Duration weeks	Effects found
Brose	RCT, community	M/F	69	3 × week 80% MC	14	36% ↑ thigh strength
Carmeli	RCT, nursing home	M/F	82	3 × week 2–5 kg weight	12	10–15% ↑ thigh strength
Charette	RCT, community	F	69	3 × week 65–75% MC	12	28–115% ↑ thigh strength, 7% ↑ type 1 fiber surface area, 20% ↑ type 2 fiber surface area
Bamman	RCT, healthy	M/F	69	3 × week 80% MC	25	82% ↑ thigh strength
Connelly	RCT, community	M/F	76	3 × week, 100% ankle dorsiflexion MC	2	15% ↑ ankle strength
Vincent	RCT, community, sedentary	M/F	68	3 × week, 50% MC 3 × week, 80% MC	24 24	16% ↑ thigh strength 20% ↑ thigh strength
Ferry	No control group Healthy and active	M	68	3 × week, 80% MC	16	27% ↑ thigh strength
Frontera	No control group Healthy and sedentary	M	60–72	3 × week, 80% MC	12	107% ↑ thigh strength
Frontera	RCT, sedentary	F	74	3 × week, 85% MC	12	39% ↑ thigh strength
Fiatarone	No control group, nursing home	M/F	90	3 × week, 80% MC	8	174% ↑ thigh strength
Fiatarone	RCT, nursing home	M/F	87	3 × week, 80% MC	10	37–178% ↑ thigh strength
Lexell	RCT, community	M/F	70–77	3 × week, 85% MC	11	163% ↑ thigh strength
Roth	RCT, community, sedentary	M/F	69	3 × week, 100% MC	13	5% ↑ thigh muscle volume

MC = Maximum capacity; ↑ = increase.

Nutritional Therapy

There are few studies on the effect of nutritional therapy on sarcopenia. Most of them have modified the protein content in the diet [21]. In a study using labeled amino acids, Volpi showed that an increase in available amino acid levels increases protein anabolism in muscle, as measured by thigh muscle biopsies. This shows that protein bioavailability is important for maintaining muscle mass, but it does not clarify the doubts regarding the efficacy of a high-protein diet in elderly patients.

Some evidence suggests that current daily protein intake recommendations (0.8 g/kg weight per day) are not sufficient enough to preserve muscle mass in the elderly. In 14 weeks, it has been shown that thigh muscle surface area decreased with this intake, as measured by CAT scan, suggesting that protein consumption should be greater.

Optimal protein intake for the elderly was recently reviewed [22]. In this review, the experts question the recommended dietary allowance for protein, 0.8 g of protein/kg per day, regardless of age. With the current evidence, we know that intake greater than the RDA can improve muscle mass, strength and function in the elderly. Therefore, in the absence of contraindications, protein intake should be about 1.5 g/kg per day.

Some studies have supplemented the diet with specific amino acids such as glutamine, leucine and other branched-chain amino acids. Branched-chain amino acids (leucine, isoleucine and valine) appear to have a significant anti-anorectic and anti-wasting effect, as they interfere with serotonin synthesis in the brain, particularly hypothalamic serotoninergic activity. Through this mechanism, they could have an anti-catabolic effect, thereby promoting protein synthesis and inhibiting intracellular proteolytic pathways. The outcome of leucine administration in young adults is beneficial, increasing fat-free mass when combined with exercise. However, fat-free mass has increased in the elderly using β-hydroxy-β-methyl butyrate (a leucine metabolite) supplementation combined with high-resistance training, but the increase in muscle strength was minimal, and not the same in all the analyzed muscle groups.

Essential amino acids have been shown to be capable of stimulating muscle protein anabolism. Positive results have been obtained by supplementing with 18 g of a combination of 10 essential amino acids, while the addition of 22 g of non-essential amino acids has not had additional impact on protein synthesis [23]. Supplementation with 8 g of a mixture of amino acids in a group of elderly patients with sarcopenia recently resulted in a significant increase in lean mass after 6 and 18 months of treatment, while also causing a reduction in plasma glucose, insulinemia and the HOMA. There was also a significant reduction in TNF-α and an increase in IGF-I levels.

Studies combining protein supplements with exercise have obtained the best outcomes when supplementation is administered immediately after exercise. The use of protein supplements without exercise, however, has not had any effect on muscle mass [18].

It is not clear whether creatine supplementation increases muscle strength in the elderly. Brose showed a substantial increase in muscle strength in a group of healthy elderly patients after 14 weeks of training with a resistance program.

Creatine administration only marginally increased the lean mass growth obtained with exercise, and muscle strength only increased with some exercises. Other longer-term studies (>4 months) show that creatine supplementation has a positive effect on muscle strength and resistance associated with resistance training programs. It is not known whether these changes last. A study was recently conducted to evaluate the effect of creatine (5 g/day) and conjugated linoleic acid (6 g/day) in a group of elderly patients subject to resistance training. Creatine supplementation increased fat-free mass and muscle strength, while the addition of conjugated linoleic acid reduced fatty mass more after 6 months of resistance training. No differences were found in isometric muscle strength.

Some studies have attempted to identify the optimal source of protein for the elderly. When comparing different isoprotein diets, the nitrogen balance is the same with either vegetable or animal proteins. However, post-absorptive protein catabolism is less inhibited with vegetable protein, resulting in less net protein synthesis. Moreover, there do appear to be differences in efficiency when 'fast' or 'slow' proteins are used, referring to the rate at which they are digested and amino acids are absorbed in the intestine. Serum protein is a rapidly absorbed soluble protein which produces a rapid, high and transient pattern of plasma amino acids, while casein is a slowly absorbed protein with a slow, more reduced and longer amino acid pattern. Protein efficiency in muscle is greater with serum protein than with casein.

Carbohydrate intake with a high glycemic index together with a mixture of proteins and amino acids just after resistance training has a positive impact on muscle protein synthesis. Other studies, however, have found a negative effect when mixing carbohydrates and amino acids in the elderly, probably due to the deregulation of the muscle protein response to insulin.

Nutritional supplementation in the elderly can have negative effects on conventional diet intake, and the final outcome can be negative [18]. It is therefore advisable to use nutrient-dense supplements that are fractioned so as not to compromise the natural diet.

Although functional improvements have been obtained with nutritional supplementation in the elderly, there are only modest increases in weight.

A relationship has recently been established between low vitamin D concentrations and high parathormone levels as risk factors for the development of sarcopenia in both male and female elderly patients. Skeletal muscle has vitamin D receptors, and a vitamin D deficiency in muscle is expressed in the form of myofibrillar degradation, a reduction in protein turnover and a hypocalcemia-induced decrease in insulin secretion. In fact, the osteomalacic myopathy described in patients with rickets improves after several weeks of vitamin D supplementation. Parathormone also has trophic effects on muscle, increasing protein metabolism.

Vitamin D deficiency is very common in the elderly and could be related to loss of muscle mass and strength. Studies with vitamin D supplementation, however, have focused more on its effect on bone mass. Some studies evaluating the fall rate in elderly patients taking vitamin D supplements found that it was lower than in non-supplemented patients, implying its positive impact on muscle mass. It therefore appears that vitamin D could help to prevent falls by improving balance. Muscle strength, walking speed and new falls were evaluated in the Frailty Intervention Trial in Elderly Subjects. After 6 months of supplementation with vitamin D or placebo, there were no differences between the two groups with regard to any of the analyzed variables. A systematic review of controlled trials to evaluate the efficacy of vitamin D supplementation on muscle strength, exercise and falls in elderly patients did not find sufficient evidence to support the use of this vitamin for these indications. Nonetheless, vitamin D supplementation has been shown to be effective in increasing bone mass and reducing falls in the elderly.

Interventions on Cytokines and Immune Function

Different strategies have been used to control the production of cytokines, which are responsible for lean mass loss in sarcopenia:

- Pentoxifylline: it reduces TNF-α messenger RNA transcription. It has helped to increase weight in other wasting models. However, there are no studies in elderly subjects.
- Thalidomide: it increases TNF-α mRNA degradation. There are no studies in the geriatric population.
- Megestrol acetate: it reduces IL-1, IL-6 and TNF-α production. Weight increases have been achieved in elderly patients with 12 weeks of treatment, together with increased intake, albumin and prealbumin levels and lymphocyte count. It has not been possible, however, to show an increase in lean mass or muscle strength.
- Omega-3 fatty acids: in animal models, they increase intake in cytokine-induced wasting processes. However, there are no studies in the elderly population.
- One new promising approach that is being investigated is the use of molecules known as angiotensin-converting enzyme inhibitors, commonly used for the treatment of hypertension. The rationale is that angiotensin II has a catabolic effect on skeletal muscle, so ACE inhibitors can delay age-related decline in muscle strength [24]. ACE inhibitors can increase the blood flow to the muscles, reducing inflammatory cytokine secretion and increasing insulin sensitivity and myocyte uptake of glucose. An increase has also been described in IGF-I and IGFBP3 levels in elderly patients with heart failure being treated with ACE inhibitors.

Possible mechanisms of action of ACE inhibitors affecting skeletal muscle include:

- Effects on cardiac function (in patients without left ventricle dysfunction):
- Increased ejection fraction
- Reduced left ventricle muscle mass
- Preserved left ventricle function
- Effects on muscular blood flow, endothelium and metabolism:
- Enhanced vascular function
- Enhanced endothelial function
- Metabolic effects:
  ° Increased serum potassium
  ° Increased IGF-I levels
  ° Increased insulin sensitivity and glucose uptake by skeletal muscle
  ° Enhanced nitric oxide production, which could increase number of sarcomeres
- Changes in type of fiber:
  ° Increase in type I figures
  ° Changes in number of mitochondria and their function
  ° Changes in skeletal muscle calcium levels
  ° Improved respiratory muscle strength
  ° Effect of ACE genotype

Recent studies suggest a close relationship between muscle strength and angiotensin-converting enzyme genotypes. Genotype II is associated with greater anabolic response to exercise, with increasingly efficient type 1 muscle fibers.

The results of intervention studies with ACE inhibitors have been contradictory thus far.

- β-Adrenergic agonists. β-Adrenergic agonists promote muscle growth by acting on the $β_2$ receptors that are predominant in skeletal muscle, thereby increasing protein synthesis and reducing catabolism. Treatment with β-adrenergic agonists, however, is limited by common (nausea, headache, insomnia) and undesirable cardiovascular effects (palpitations, increased risk of ischemia, heart failure, arrhythmia and sudden death). New agonists have been tested, including formoterol, which can induce an anabolic response in skeletal muscle at low doses, with few effects on the heart and cardiovascular system when compared with classic β-adrenergic agents (fenoterol, clenbuterol).

References

1 Elia M, Zellipour L, Stratton R: To screen or not to screen for adult malnutrition. Clin Nutr 2005;24:867–884.

2 Cruz-Jentoft A, Baeyens JP, Bauer JM, et al: Sarcopenia: European consensus on definition and diagnosis. Report of the European Working Group on Sarcopenia in Older People. Age Ageing 2010;39:412–423.

Burgos Peláez

3   Doherty TJ: Aging and sarcopenia. J Appl Physiol 2003;95:1717–1727.

4   Marcell TJ: Sarcopenia: causes, consequences and preventions. J Gerontol A Biol Sci Med Sci 2003;58:911–916.

5   Hebuterne X, Bermon S, Schneider SM: Ageing and muscle: the effects of malnutrition, re-nutrition and physical exercise. Curr Opin Clin Nutr Metab Care 2001;4:295–300.

6   Hughes VA, Frontera WR, Roubenoff R, et al: Longitudinal changes in body composition in older men and women: role of body weight change and physical activity. Am J Clin Nutr 2002;76:473–481.

7   Borst SE: Interventions for sarcopenia and muscle weakness in older people. Age Ageing 2004;33:548–555.

8   Lynch GS, Schertzer JD, Ryall JG: Therapeutic approaches for muscle wasting disorders. Pharmacol Ther 2007;113:461–487.

9   Waters DL, Baumgartner RN, Garry PJ: Advantages of dietary, exercise-related, and therapeutic options to prevent and treat sarcopenia in older adult patients: an update. Clin Interv Aging 2010;5:259–270.

10 Bhasin S: Testosterone supplementation for aging-associated sarcopenia. J Gerontol A Biol Sci Med Sci 2003;58:1002–1008.

11 Percheron G, Hogrel JY, Denot-Ledunois S: Effect of 1-year oral administration of dehydroepiandrosterone to 60- to 80-year-old individuals on muscle function and cross-sectional area: a double-blind placebo-controlled trial. Arch Intern Med 2003;163:720–727.

12 Bross R, Javanbakht M, Bhasin S: Anabolic interventions for aging-associated sarcopenia. J Clin Endocrinol Metab 1999;84:3420–3430.

13 Kenny AM, Dawson L, Kleppinger A, et al: Prevalence of sarcopenia and predictors of skeletal muscle mass in non-obese women who are long-term users of estrogen replacement therapy. J Gerontol A Biol Sci Med Sci 2003;58A:436–440.

14 Svensson J, Stibrant Sunnerhagen KS, Johannsson G: Five years of growth hormone replacement therapy in adults: age- and gender-related changes in isometric and isokinetic muscle strength. J Clin Endocrinol Metab 2003;88:2061–2069.

15 Giovannini S, Marzetti E, Borst SE, Leeuwenburgh C: Modulation of GH/IGF-1 axis: potential strategies to counteract sarcopenia in older adults. Mech Ageing Dev DOI: 10.1016/j.mad.2008.08.001.

16 Latham NK, Bennett DA, Stretton CM, Anderson CS: Systematic review of progressive resistance strength training in older adults. J Gerontol A Biol Sci Med Sci 2004;59:48–61.

17 Yarasheski KE: Exercise, aging and muscle protein metabolism. J Gerontol A Biol Sci Med Sci 2003;58:918–922.

18 Fiatarone MA, O'Neill EF, Ryan ND, et al: Exercise training and nutritional supplementation for physical frailty in very elderly people. N Engl J Med 1994;330:1769–1775.

19 Paddon-Jones D, Short KR, Campbell WW, et al: Role of dietary protein in the sarcopenia of aging. Am J Clin Nutr 2008;87(suppl):1562S–1566S.

20 Campbell WW, Leidy HJ: Dietary protein and resistance training effects on muscle and body composition in older persons.

21 Dreyer HC, Volpi E: Role of protein and amino acids in the pathophysiology and treatment of sarcopenia. J Am Col Nutr 2005;24:140S–145S.

22 Wolfe R, Miller S, Miller K: Optimal protein intake in the elderly. Clin Nutr 2008;27:675–684.

23 Volpi E, Kobayashi H, Sheffield-Moore M, et al: Essential amino acids are primarily responsible for the amino acid stimulation of muscle protein anabolism in healthy elderly adults. Am J Clin Nutr 2003;78:250–258.

24 Sumukadas D, Witham MD, Struthers AD, Mcmurdo MET: ACE inhibitors as a therapy for sarcopenia-evidence and possible mechanisms. J Nutr 2008;12:480–485.

Interventions

Cichero J, Clavé P (eds): Stepping Stones to Living Well with Dysphagia.
Nestlé Nutr Inst Workshop Ser, vol 72, pp 101–108,
Nestec Ltd., Vevey/S. Karger AG., Basel, © 2012

Importance of Nutritional Support in Older People

E. Sánchez García · B. Montero Errasquín ·
C. Sánchez Castellano · A.J. Cruz-Jentoft

Servicio de Geriatría, Hospital Universitario Ramón y Cajal, Madrid, Spain

Abstract

Proper nutrition is an essential part of successful aging and may delay the onset of diseases. Nutrition-related problems in older subjects have been long-time ignored; good nutritional status is an essential component of health and a relevant part of therapeutic plans of most chronic diseases. Moreover, food and nutrition are a relevant aspect of most cultures and are strongly linked with individual lifestyles. Research has proved that nutritional intervention can improve outcomes in many clinical scenarios. This is especially true for older individuals with different acute and chronic conditions and diseases, or with malnutrition. Nutritional intervention can provide sufficient energy, protein and micronutrients, maintain or improve nutritional status, reduce morbidity and increase survival. Evidence is still lacking on the impact of nutritional intervention on physical and mental function, and on quality of life, very relevant outcomes for older individuals. Nutritional screening and assessment should become part of health care of both healthy and sick older people. Nutritional counseling and intervention should be embedded in a general care plan that takes into account all aspects of an aging person. Nutritional programs that aim for high compliance should be individualized, and would have to consider every aspect of old age: beliefs, attitudes, preferences, expectations, and aspirations.

Copyright © 2012 Nestec Ltd., Vevey/S. Karger AG, Basel

Life expectancy has been increasing in developed countries over the past two centuries at a pace that makes some experts suggest that most babies born in the first decade of the XXI century in developed countries will celebrate their 100th birthdays [1].

Populations of these countries are ageing fast for many reasons, and research suggests that ageing processes may be amenable to modification, with a postponement of functional limitations.

Nutrition and Successful Aging

Proper nutrition is an essential part of successful aging, and may delay the onset of diseases. Although improvement of health and functional trajectories along life depends mostly on improvements in older people, this process should probably start by improving living conditions and lifestyle earlier in life. Progress towards improvement of health is likely to depend on public health to combat many problems, inadequate nutrition being a major area of improvement [2, 3]. Good nutrition and physical exercise are essential for healthy ageing from both a physical and psychological perspective. Therefore, a multidisciplinary life course approach to ageing is vital to minimizing its complications for quality of life and subsequent public health [4].

Nutrition-related problems in older subjects, formerly ignored, have been gaining prominence in recent years and are now highly relevant, both in research and in usual clinical practice. Having a good nutritional status is not only linked to health and welfare, but is also related to an increased life expectancy with reduced disability, and is an essential component of the therapeutic plan in most chronic diseases. Moreover, food and nutrition is a relevant aspect of most cultures and is related with the individual lifestyle of every person [5].

If good nutrition is key for healthy aging, nutritional assessment and intervention should become part of health care of both healthy and sick older people. Nutritional counseling and intervention should be part of a general care plan that takes into account all aspects of an aging person. The promotion of health in older individuals should incorporate the principles of Gerontology and Geriatric Medicine to public health interventions. At individual level, strategies of successful ageing consist of having the opportunity to make and making healthy lifestyle choices, implementing various self-management techniques. Nutritional programs that aim for high compliance should be individualized, and would have to consider every aspect of old age: beliefs, attitudes, preferences, expectations, and aspirations [6].

It is now scientific evidence that older people cannot be understood with the same parameters as younger adults: ageing and many prevalent diseases in old age change nutritional needs along lifetime. Thus, specific guidelines on nutrition and recommended intakes for older adults have been released in the last decades by several organizations. However, variability of most parameters also increases with age, making older individuals an extremely heterogeneous population, with specific needs for each individual. Even laypersons can acknowledge that a healthy and active octogenarian will not have the same needs and demands as a frail octogenarian with multiple disabling comorbidities and polypharmacy. Thus, in the near future, special recommendations for subgroups of individuals are essential, taking into account individual health status and other factors [7].

Sánchez García · Montero Errasquín · Sánchez Castellano · Cruz-Jentoft

The Imperative of Detecting and Treating Malnutrition in Older Subjects

Medicine is unable to cure most chronic diseases nowadays, but is able to prolong life in those who suffer chronic conditions. When diseases appear, nutritional intervention may increase survival and improve health outcomes for many diseases. Therefore, regular nutritional screening and assessment is recommended in older subjects – especially in the frailest and in specific care settings (hospitals, nursing homes) to early identify nutritional problems and start a rapid nutritional intervention before malnutrition impairs health status [8]. When malnutrition is detected, a search for the underlying diagnosis is mandatory in order to set up the optimal management strategy [9]. Unfortunately, systematic nutritional screening and assessment programs are still underdeveloped, both in the community and in specific settings where nutritional problems are highly prevalent (hospital, nursing homes). The extension of these programs is financially sound, as intervention on individuals at risk of malnutrition should be much cheaper than interventions in undernourished patients, although this will have to be better proved [10, 11].

Nutritional science has academically developed fast in recent years. Nutrition being an essential aspect of health, it is surprising how little attention has been paid to this discipline, both in universities and in usual clinical practice. Many physicians lack nutritional literacy and have not incorporated nutrition in their view of complex or chronic patients [12]. However, sound research on nutritional intervention has proved that nutritional intervention, usually in the form of oral supplements or tube feeding, can improve outcomes in many diseases [13]. This is true for older individuals: those admitted for surgery of a fractured hip, gastrointestinal surgery, stroke, chronic liver disease, lung diseases and many other prevalent chronic conditions will benefit from a structured nutritional intervention. In fact, the best evidence available favors nutritional intervention in older individuals.

Malnutrition is one of the first geriatric syndromes ('geriatric giants'), and is linked, through sarcopenia, to impaired health outcomes and increased health care costs [13]. Malnutrition has deleterious effects on the recovery and well-being of a wide range of patients and diseases. The goal of nutritional support is to fight malnutrition by supplying all nutrients required for the energy, plastic, and regulatory needs of a given individual, aiming to maintain or restore the functional integrity of the body, including nutritional status, physical and mental function, and quality of life, and to reduce morbidity and mortality.

Effectiveness of Nutritional Intervention

Evidence on the effectiveness of nutritional support in complying with this is growing. At present, nutritional intervention can provide sufficient energy, protein and micronutrients, maintain or improve nutritional status, reduce morbidity and increase survival, especially in undernourished individuals [14]. Unfortunately, evidence is not so strong on the impact of nutritional intervention on physical and mental function, and on quality of life, very relevant outcomes for older individuals. More research is needed in this area.

Recent guidelines on nutritional intervention in older people have shown some specific situations where nutritional intervention may have a role [14]. Very unfortunately, health authorities in most countries still consider nutrition as something which is unrelated to health status and outcomes, and most European countries still do not have wide range nutritional screening programs, and do not pay for nutritional intervention. This is not in the best interest of frail older citizens, or of tax payers, who are paying for health consequences that may be preventable with a small investment, as nutritional interventions are usually cost effective [15, 16]. It is still surprising how resources are easily allocated to very expensive areas of health care (cancer, aids, transplantation) to benefit a limited number of citizens, and are restricted in areas that involve wellbeing of a high number of citizens – being the desire of most people not to die before old age comes. This may be only another face of an old problem – named ageism [17].

As mentioned before, strong evidence supports the implementation of nutritional intervention in some clinical scenarios. We will review two of them that are very well established and are good examples of the principles mentioned above: older patients with malnutrition, and older patients with dysphagia.

Nutritional Intervention Is Medical Care

Malnutrition (undernutrition) is a complex geriatric syndrome that leads to impaired health and functional outcomes, including a high risk of short-term mortality. Hunger is still a major cause of mortality at all ages in many areas of the world. Malnutrition is also a well-known marker of severity of other diseases. Although this fact seems underrecognized, malnutrition is still frequent nowadays in developed countries, where it clusters in older individuals rather than in children. The global prevalence of malnutrition in older individuals is estimated at 22.8%, with considerable differences between care settings (rehabilitation, 50.5%; hospital, 38.7%; nursing home, 13.8%; community, 5.8%) [18].

Treatment of malnutrition includes addressing the causes that lead into it, and correcting any deficit in macro- and micronutrient intake and status. Thus, symptomatic (as opposed to etiological) treatment of malnutrition requires an intervention in nutrient intake to improve nutritional status. Laypersons, political decision makers, and even some health care professionals sometimes suggest that this intervention will always be successful by making changes in the usual food that individuals eat, and thus do not consider that nutritional treatment

Sánchez García · Montero Errasquín · Sánchez Castellano · Cruz-Jentoft

of malnutrition is a medical intervention. Although this may be true in some cases, this is an oversimplistic view of a major clinical problem. To be successful, treatment of malnourished patients needs a specific nutritional intervention, carefully tailored, implemented and followed by well-trained health care providers.

Enteral nutrition (oral supplements or tube feeding) plays a major role in such patients. Oral nutritional supplementation has shown clear benefits in older malnourished patients by increasing energy, protein and micronutrient intake, maintaining or improving nutritional status and increasing survival [14]. Positive effects of oral supplements for up to 18 months have been confirmed in a Cochrane meta-analysis that included 62 trials with 10,187 randomized participants. Maximum duration of intervention was 18 months. Mortality was reduced when participants were defined as undernourished (RR 0.79) [19]. Benefits were most relevant in those subjects older than 75 years.

Nutritional support should be started as soon as a problem is detected. Although evidence suggests that enteral nutrition is mostly beneficial in undernourished individuals, usual medical practice for many severe diseases shows that prevention or early intervention may be more efficient. Thus, identifying individuals at high risk of undernutrition (to prevent them running into it by the right intervention) or when malnutrition is starting seems to be a sound strategy that will have to be better tested in clinical trials.

Nutritional Intervention in Dysphagia

Dysphagia is a major problem in Geriatric Medicine, where swallowing problems sum up with age-related changes in swallowing function [20]. Prevalence of dysphagia increases with age. The most frequent etiologies of dysphagia in old age are neurological diseases (i.e. stroke, Parkinson's disease and dementias, including Alzheimer's disease). Other conditions that may cause dysphagia in this population are dysfunctions of the upper esophageal sphincter, including cricopharyngeal achalasia, Zenker diverticula or cancer.

Complications of dysphagia depend on its severity. When swallowing is ineffective, malnutrition and dehydration will follow, with progressive loss of muscle mass (sarcopenia, physical dependency), changes in the immune system (immune suppression, infections) and wound healing problems (pressure ulcers). If swallowing is unsafe, aspiration may follow – a dreaded but frequent problem in acute care settings. All these complications are associated with increased hospital stays, higher costs of care, and increased mortality. Psychosocial consequences of dysphagia also have a major impact on quality of life, as feeding is a social and cultural event. Thus, assessment of the nutritional status of older patients with dysphagia should be mandatory for clinicians and dietitians, and regular monitoring of nutritional status may prevent, detect early and allow intervention before complications arise. Many other chapters in this publication are devoted to different aspects of the management of dysphagia.

Dysphagia, for the purposes of this chapter, serves as a model of malnutrition secondary to a specific etiology, and the relevance of early starting nutritional support in dysphagia patients will be emphasized. Generally speaking, nutritional intervention in older patients with swallowing problems must be comprehensive, and has to provide the right daily individual needs of macronutrients (energy, protein, fat and carbohydrates), fiber, minerals, vitamins and water to maintain a healthy nutritional status, following usual recommendations on healthy diet for people over 70 years. Feeding should be safe, which is usually feasible by making the right changes in food texture and quantity, sometimes with the help of supplements and thickeners. And the pleasure and social aspects of eating must also be taken into account by adjusting food presentation, colors, forms, and aromas to fit personal preferences and tastes, always fighting monotony.

Dysphagia is one of the most prevalent conditions that limit food intake in older individuals, and neurological causes of dysphagia rank first in this population. It is not surprising to learn that many clinical intervention studies have been performed in such patients. In dysphagia of neurological origin, nutritional intervention depends on the type and extent of the swallowing disturbance. Nutritional intervention should be associated with intensive swallowing therapy with the aim of recovering safe and sufficient oral intake.

In geriatric patients with severe neurologic dysphagia, strong evidence supports the use of enteral nutrition to maintain or improve nutritional status [14]. Nutritional therapy includes a wide range of interventions, from minor changes in normal diet, through the modification of food consistency or the use of thickeners, to total enteral nutrition administered by a nasoenteric tube or a gastrostomy. As neurological dysphagia may change with time, any treatment must be individualized and regularly adapted with time.

Clinical trials in acute stroke with dysphagia are difficult to perform and interpret, as not offering nutritional support in acute stroke (i.e. having a non-intervention control group) is unacceptable from an ethical point of view. Stroke patients with severe dysphagia will be unable to safely eat by mouth, sometimes for prolonged periods of time, and using artificial nutrition in such patients is standard care, at least for some time, to warrant nutrient intake and avoid complications of malnutrition.

There are open questions on the best way to feed (is gastrostomy better than enteral tubes?) and on how early in the course of the disease should nutritional intervention be started. This latest point is important, as dysphagia may be reversible in stroke patients. Some studies on the natural course of dysphagia after stroke show that spontaneous remission happens at 7–14 days after the acute event in 73–86% of cases [21]. When dysphagia persists after 2 weeks,

Sánchez García · Montero Errasquín · Sánchez Castellano · Cruz-Jentoft

some extra 4–29% of patients recover the ability to eat by mouth in a period that ranges from 4 to 31 months.

At this time, clinical guidelines recommend to start enteral nutrition immediately after stroke in geriatric patients with severe neurological dysphagia [14], when there is no clear reason not to do so. Early nutrition seems to improve survival, reduce length of hospital stay and improve functional status in these patients, especially in older patients, but not all studies have confirmed this. An old Cochrane review of nutritional interventions for dysphagia in acute stroke concluded that enteral nutrition using a gastrostomy could be associated with better nutritional outcomes, but the evidence is weak [22, 23].

Dysphagia and other nutritional problems in the setting of advanced neurodegenerative diseases (usually Parkinson's or Alzheimer's disease) are more complex, and evidence is lacking to guide clinical practice in these patients [14, 24]. Enteral feeding or nutritional supplements can improve nutritional status of patients with dementia, at least in mild to moderate stages, and nutritional status is linked to the development of dementia. In advanced dementia, values and preferences play a major role, and the decision should be individualized.

References

1   Christensen K, Doblhammer G, Rau R, et al: Ageing populations: the challenges ahead. Lancet 2009;374:1196–1208.

2   Riley J: Rising Life Expectancy: A Global History. New York, Cambridge University Press, 2001.

3   McKeown RE: The Epidemiologic Transition: Changing Patterns of Mortality and Population Dynamics. Am J Lifestyle Med 2009;3:19S–26S.

4   Shepherd A: Nutrition through the life span. Part 3: adults aged 65 years and over. Br J Nurs 2009;18:301–302, 304–307.

5   Woo J: Nutritional strategies for successful aging. Med Clin North Am 2011;95:477–493, ix–x.

6   Cruz-Jentoft A, Franco A, Sommer P, et al: European silver paper on the future of health promotion and preventive actions, basic research, and clinical aspects of age-related disease. Eur J Ageing 2009;6:51–57.

7   Cannella C, Savina C, Donini LM: Nutrition, longevity and behavior. Arch Gerontol Geriatr 2009;49(suppl 1):19–27.

8   Kondrup J, Allison SP, Elia M, et al: ESPEN guidelines for nutrition screening 2002. Clin Nutr 2003;22:415–421.

9   Jensen GL, Mirtallo J, Compher C, et al: Adult starvation and disease-related malnutrition: a proposal for etiology-based diagnosis in the clinical practice setting from the International Consensus Guideline Committee. JPEN J Parenter Enteral Nutr 2010;34:156–159.

10 Olveira G, Tapia MJ, Colomo N: Costs versus benefits of oral nutritional supplements (in Spanish). Nutr Hosp 2009;24:251–259.

11 Elia M, Russell CA, Stratton RJ: Malnutrition in the UK: policies to address the problem. Proc Nutr Soc 2010;69:470–476.

12 Lindorff-Larsen K, Hojgaard Rasmussen H, Kondrup J, et al: Management and perception of hospital undernutrition – a positive change among Danish doctors and nurses. Clin Nutr 2007;26:371–378.

13 Cruz-Jentoft AJ, Landi F, Topinkova E, et al: Understanding sarcopenia as a geriatric syndrome. Curr Opin Clin Nutr Metab Care 2010;13:1–7.

14 Volkert D, Berner YN, Berry E, et al: ESPEN Guidelines on Enteral Nutrition: Geriatrics. Clin Nutr 2006;25:330–360.

15 Guest JF, Panca M, Baeyens JP, et al: Health economic impact of managing patients following a community-based diagnosis of malnutrition in the UK. Clin Nutr 2011;30:422–429.

16 Freijer K, Nuijten MJ: Analysis of the health economic impact of medical nutrition in the Netherlands. Eur J Clin Nutr 2010;64:1229–1234.

17 Butler RN: Age-ism: another form of bigotry. Gerontologist 1969;9:243–246.

18 Kaiser MJ, Bauer JM, Ramsch C, et al: Frequency of malnutrition in older adults: a multinational perspective using the mini nutritional assessment. J Am Geriatr Soc 2010;58:1734–1738.

19 Milne AC, Potter J, Vivanti A, et al: Protein and energy supplementation in elderly people at risk from malnutrition. Cochrane Database Syst Rev 2009;2:CD003288.

20 Ney DM, Weiss JM, Kind AJ, et al: Senescent swallowing: impact, strategies, and interventions. Nutr Clin Pract 2009;24:395–413.

21 Smithard DG, O'Neill PA, England RE, et al: The natural history of dysphagia following a stroke. Dysphagia 1997;12:188–193.

22 Bath PM, Bath FJ, Smithard DG: Interventions for dysphagia in acute stroke. Cochrane Database Syst Rev 2000;CD000323.

23 Foley N, Teasell R, Salter K, et al: Dysphagia treatment post stroke: a systematic review of randomised controlled trials. Age Ageing 2008;37:258–264.

24 Sampson EL, Candy B, Jones L: Enteral tube feeding for older people with advanced dementia. Cochrane Database Syst Rev 2009;CD007209.

Cichero J, Clavé P (eds): Stepping Stones to Living Well with Dysphagia.
Nestlé Nutr Inst Workshop Ser, vol 72, pp 109–117,
Nestec Ltd., Vevey/S. Karger AG., Basel, © 2012

Exercise-Based Approaches to Dysphagia Rehabilitation

Catriona M. Steele

Toronto Rehabilitation Institute, University of Toronto, and Bloorview Research Institute, Toronto, ON, Canada

Abstract

Rehabilitative techniques for dysphagia (swallowing impairment) increasingly employ exercise modeled on methods used to train muscles in sports medicine. Three techniques in particular show promise for improving muscle strength and function related to swallowing: the Shaker exercise, expiratory muscle strength training, and tongue pressure resistance training. All three techniques invoke principles of task specificity, muscular load, resistance, and intensity, and aim to achieve functional changes in swallowing through changes in muscle physiology derived from strength or endurance training. To date, studies of treatment benefit arising from these techniques involve small sample sizes; this is particularly true of randomized studies with controls receiving standard treatment or experiencing spontaneous recovery. Nevertheless, a review of the available literature shows that improvement of penetration-aspiration is a common finding for individuals with dysphagia receiving one of these three treatment approaches. Although hypothesized as an expected outcome of swallow muscle strength training, improvements in post-swallow residues are noted to be uncommon as an outcome of these exercise-based approaches. The available evidence suggests that exercise-based approaches to swallowing rehabilitation do succeed in changing muscle strength and function, but generalization to true swallowing tasks may be somewhat limited.

The field of dysphagia diagnosis and intervention is relatively young, with current practices dating back to the pioneering work of Logemann, whose first textbook was published in 1983 [1]. Prior to the publication of that book, the dysphagia literature was dominated by studies profiling swallowing impairment seen in a variety of specific etiologies, and by descriptions of protocols for the radiological examination of swallowing function. Beginning in the 1980s, studies describing techniques for dysphagia intervention emerged. These early techniques fell exclusively into the category of compensatory interventions, that is, interventions that are intended to yield an immediate but transient improvement in swallowing function, provided that the technique is used correctly. Examples of compensatory interventions include the use of thickened liquids and food texture modifications to manipulate the flow of material through the pharynx. Other compensatory interventions are behavioral techniques that must be learned by the patient. Postural modifications such as chin down or head turn are intended to change the configuration of the oropharynx so that the bolus can be contained in the mouth without spilling, collects in the vallecular space in the case of spillage, and flows effectively through the hypopharynx and upper esophageal sphincter (UES). Different postures are indicated for different types of impairment; for example, a head turn is described to direct the bolus away from the side of weakness in a patient with unilateral pharyngeal paresis, thereby utilizing the stronger and intact muscles on the unimpaired side [2]. Other behavioral techniques involve volitional efforts to enhance airway closure or hyolaryngeal excursion, such as the supraglottic swallow and the Mendelsohn maneuver. A final class of compensatory interventions involves stimulation techniques, intended to heighten sensory input and evoke a more timely and effective swallow motor response. Thermal tactile stimulation is probably the best known of these techniques, described to yield improvements in swallow transit times, but subsequently shown to have only a transient, time-limited effect [3–5]. Later studies exploring other modalities of stimulation, such as taste, have shown similar, transient effects [6].

Around the mid-1990s, discussions emerge in the literature regarding the possibility that some dysphagia interventions might have the potential for longer-lasting effects, i.e. to effect permanent changes in swallowing physiology. These techniques became known as *rehabilitative interventions* and were described as 'interventions that, when provided *over the course of time*, are thought to result in *permanent* changes in the substrates underlying deglutition; i.e., *changing the physiology* of the swallowing mechanism' [7]. An important distinction regarding rehabilitative interventions is that it is intended that the patient will not need to remember to use the technique whenever they swallow. The goal is to restore functional swallowing that does not require compensation.

A number of the previously described compensatory interventions have been recognized to have possible rehabilitative potential, if practiced in a rigorous and repetitive manner. Stimulation techniques including thermal, electrical, air pulse and transcranial magnetic methods are currently under investigation for their potential to elicit neuroplastic changes in swallowing motor control [8–13]. With respect to behavioral techniques, Kahrilas et al. [14, 15] describe a patient who learned to use the Mendelsohn maneuver to overcome difficulties in UES opening and regained swallowing function. Similar stories were reported for case series of patients with long-standing pharyngeal and UES impairment by Crary et al. [16, 17] and Huckabee and Cannito [18]. These studies were among the first to train patients to perform swallowing exercises over the course of at least 10 treatment sessions, scheduled regularly (i.e. daily or twice daily), and involving multiple task repetitions within each treatment session. Such protocols resemble the kinds of exercise regimens used in the gym for cardiac fitness, muscle strengthening or weight loss training. That is, they involve many repetitions of a task, ideally performed at a difficulty level that will lead either to skilled task performance through learning and/or to changes in the muscles that are challenged during the task. However, it is known that changes in muscle tone, strength and bulk are unlikely to be achieved without consideration of exercise load, resistance, intensity and duration. Burkhead et al. [19] argues that similar considerations need to be applied to rehabilitative swallowing exercises.

Several different examples of swallowing interventions are candidates for use in an exercise-based protocol. Some have been studied, showing proof-of-principle that repeated practice over a 6–8-week time frame can indeed lead to changes in swallowing physiology. For example, the Shaker exercise is a head-lifting technique performed in the supine position, and intended to specifically exercise the suprahyoid muscles. Gravity provides a source of fixed resistance, and the exercise is performed in both an isometric (sustained) and isokinetic (short repetitions) manner [20]. The Shaker exercise is indicated for patients who display impaired UES opening, given the recognition that excursion of the hyolaryngeal complex is biomechanically linked to UES opening. By improving the strength of the muscles responsible for superior and anterior hyolaryngeal excursion in swallowing, the technique aims to facilitate greater UES opening and reduced UES pressures. Preliminary data from healthy adults who practiced this technique support these hypotheses, as do results from patients who have performed the Shaker exercise compared to those performing a sham exercise [20, 21]. Penetration-aspiration has also been reported to improve in these patients.

A second example of an exercise-based approach to dysphagia intervention is expiratory muscle strength training (EMST), originally developed for patients with respiratory difficulties and voice disorders [22]. Patients are required to do forced exhalation through a device that provides resistance to expiratory airflow. Varying degrees of resistance can be set in the device, and patients are instructed to do 20 min of practice daily over 4 weeks. Early work with this exercise suggested that the suprahyoid muscles become engaged during expiratory threshold training tasks [23], lending support to the idea that the technique might have benefits for swallowing. Two recent studies in individuals with Parkinson's disease have shown improvements in penetration-aspiration and in hyoid movement following 4 weeks of EMST [24, 25].

Perhaps the most-studied form of exercise training for dysphagia is resistance training for the tongue. The rationale for strength training of the tongue dates back to studies documenting reduced pressures on maximum isometric tongue-palate press tasks in healthy older adults [26]. An important point about these findings is that age-related declines are not seen in swallowing pressures, which utilize less than half of each person's maximum tongue pressure capacity. Nevertheless, given the observation of reduced maximum tongue pressures and other literature suggesting atrophy in tongue and neck muscles similar to that seen in sarcopenia of the leg muscles, Robbins et al. [27] designed an 8-week program of repetitive tongue pressure resistance exercise. In this program, participants perform 60 tongue-palate presses each day, on alternate days of the week, for a total of 24 sessions over 8 weeks. The exercises in each session are distributed evenly between anterior and posterior tongue-palate presses, and an important component of the program is the identification of a target work zone, or load, for each patient, between 60 and 80% of their maximum capacity. Repeated measurement of maximum capacity each week allows for incremental super-stepping of the target zone. Healthy seniors who followed this regimen showed a 20% increase in maximum isometric pressures versus baseline [27]. This provided the preliminary evidence to justify application of the technique in patients with dysphagia.

In 2007, Robbins et al. [28] published the results of a preliminary case series study of tongue pressure resistance training in stroke patients with dysphagia. These individuals were described to have an average penetration-aspiration scale score of 6 (aspiration below the true vocal folds) on 10-ml swallows of thin liquid barium at baseline, and their maximum isometric tongue pressures fell below 40 kPa – the range reported to be normal for older men. After 8 weeks of tongue pressure resistance training, pressure capacity had increased by 46% for anterior-, and by a dramatic 81% for posterior-emphasis tasks. Importantly, penetration-aspiration scale scores also improved in this group, with the post-treatment mean falling at 1 (i.e. no penetration or aspiration). Robbins et al. [28] also monitored other components of swallowing function in videofluoroscopy. Despite the improvement in penetration-aspiration, no systematic improvements in residue were observed in this patient group. It should be recognized that these patients, who were in the first 6 months following stroke, may have enjoyed some spontaneous recovery. The degree to which the treatment may be responsible for the observed improvements is unclear.

In our lab at the Toronto Rehabilitation Institute we have been interested in tongue pressure resistance training, but challenged by the data showing that swallowing is a task that does not utilize a person's full tongue pressure capacity. We have been particularly interested in the role played by the tongue in controlling thin liquid bolus flow, and speculated that this requires a precise matching of applied tongue pressure to the inherent viscosity or flow characteristics of a bolus in order to achieve the desired result. Our prior work in studying tongue movements and tongue pressure generation in swallowing strongly suggests that tongue pressures build during the time when the body of the tongue is raised and pressing forward along the palate [29]. These anterior-superior pressures

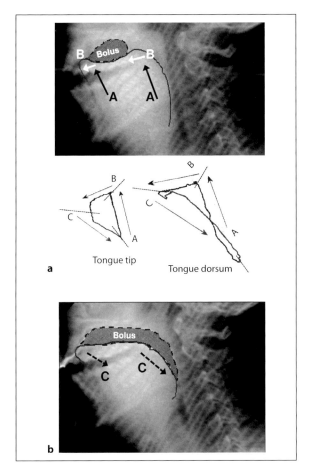

Fig. 1. **a** Pressure rise. The bolus is compressed between tongue and palate. The tongue squeezes forward under bolus. Viscosity (resistance to flow) is detected as the bolus is subjected to shearing forces. Path of tongue movement: A = anterior-superior (initial pressure rise); B = anterior (continued pressure rise and bolus squeezing); C = posterior-inferior (pressure release). **b** Pressure release. The posterior tongue lowers; pressure release allows the bolus to flow. Bolus flow evolves as a function of liquid viscosity and tongue pressure release slope: (amplitude/duration).

are thought to generate squeezing forces that move liquid boluses backwards through the mouth towards the pharynx (fig. 1). In cases where insufficient pressure is applied, particularly by the back of the tongue, it seems likely that a very low-viscosity liquid will spill into the pharynx under its own inertia. A thicker consistency might not be effectively propelled, leaving oral and pharyngeal residues.

Based on these ideas, we hypothesized that the ability to achieve precise pressures, and to vary pressures to match bolus viscosity, might be important for bolus control. The analogy here is that the tongue might be doing something similar to what the hand and arm do, when trying to manage to balance an upright pole without it falling, except that in the case of swallowing, the task requires both balancing and transporting the liquid bolus in a controlled manner. Therefore, we designed a modification to the Robbins protocol, in which the target zone for practice involved a series of variable pressure targets, falling between 20 and 90% of the patient's maximum values. The task is analogous to hitting a series of different bull's-eye targets precisely with darts, rather than lifting incrementally heavier weights. In practice, this involves the speech-language pathologist measuring maximum pressure capacity across a series of 5 maximum isometric pressures at the beginning of the treatment session (e.g. mean of 30 kPa), and then randomly choosing submaximal values, which the patient tries to generate with accuracy (e.g. 15, 22, 27, etc.) during therapy. Feedback regarding accuracy in reaching the target pressure without overshoot or undershoot can be provided based on pressure amplitude readings on hand-held manometers such as the Iowa Oral Performance Instrument. As in the Robbins protocol, each treatment session involves 60 tongue pressure training tasks, distributed equally between those emphasizing anterior tongue-palate pressure and posterior tongue-palate pressures.

Our first 3 patients demonstrated different patterns of change with this treatment, described in a previous publication [30]. One patient, within 6 months after cortical stroke, showed rapid gains in maximum strength across the first 12 sessions of treatment, and then plateaued. Another patient, 4 years after skull base tumor resection, in which the hypoglossal nerve sustained iatrogenic injury, showed very little change in the first 12 sessions of treatment, but then showed rapid gains from session 12 to 24. This pattern suggests that individuals with chronic injury may require longer courses of treatment in order to respond. A third patient, 4 years after brainstem hemorrhage, showed no change in tongue pressure capacity across 24 sessions of treatment, but elected to continue training, with remote monitoring, for a total of 1 year (138 sessions) of treatment. He showed very slow improvement, but eventually reached a maximum isometric tongue pressure of 40 kPa around session 90, showing further gains beyond that point, as illustrated in figure 2. The obvious tongue weakness and slow initial recovery in this patient may be partially attributable to a Botox injection that had been administered to his submandibular area in order to limit oral secretions; this injection contributed to increased dysarthria and may, therefore, have impacted his tongue muscles. However, our data suggest that even with chronic atrophy and putative neurotoxin-induced peripheral injury, tongue pressure resistance training can be used to build tongue muscle strength and pressure generation capacity. Such gains appear to be seen both when treatment emphasizes strength targets between 60 and 80% of maximum and when the emphasis is placed on variable pressure accuracy between 20 and 90% of maximum.

Following these early pilot results, we have continued to investigate tongue pressure strength and accuracy training in individuals with neurogenic

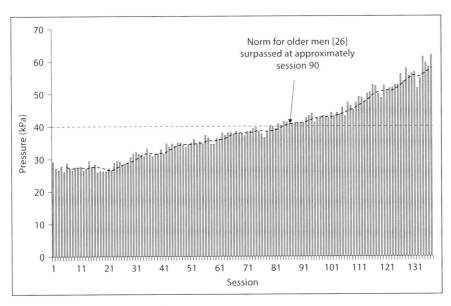

Fig. 2. Anterior tongue strength.

dysphagia. We have worked with an etiologically heterogeneous group including patients with dysphagia following stroke, acquired brain injury, or skull base tumor resection, and also with frail elders with neurologic conditions like Parkinson's disease. The common thread among these individuals has been evidence of poor oral bolus containment with thin liquids on videofluoroscopy. We have conducted a controlled case series in individuals who have all completed 24 sessions of treatment with pre- and posttreatment videofluoroscopy. Results of that study are currently in the process of publication, but demonstrate similar findings to those of Robbins et al. [28], namely improvements in penetration-aspiration scale scores with thin liquid stimuli, but no systematic improvements in pharyngeal residues with spoon-thick stimuli.

The persistence of pharyngeal residues following all three of the different approaches to exercise-based dysphagia intervention that we have reviewed (Shaker exercise, EMST, tongue pressure resistance training) suggests that we have not yet found treatment tasks that have adequate specificity for the process of pharyngeal bolus clearance.

In conclusion, exercise-based interventions require careful design, with attention to task selection and specificity, load, intensity and treatment duration. To date, there is preliminary evidence that penetration-aspiration can be reduced through exercise-based interventions in neurogenic dysphagia.

References

1 Logemann JA: Evaluation and Treatment of Swallowing Disorders, ed 2. San Diego, College Hill Press, 1997.

2 Rasley A, Logemann JA, Kahrilas PJ, et al: Prevention of barium aspiration during videofluoroscopic swallowing studies: value of change in posture. AJR Am J Roentgenol 1993;160:1005–1009.

3 Lazzara G, Lazarus C, Logemann JA: Impact of thermal stimulation on the triggering of the swallowing reflex. Dysphagia 1986;1:73–77.

4 Rosenbek J, Roecker EB, Wood JL, Robbins J: Thermal application reduces the duration of stage transition in dysphagia after stroke. Dysphagia 1996;11:4.

5 Rosenbek JC, Robbins J, Fishback B, Levine RL: Effects of thermal application on dysphagia after stroke. J Speech Hear Res 1991;34:1257–1268.

6 Sciortino K, Liss JM, Case JL, et al: Effects of mechanical, cold, gustatory, and combined stimulation to the human anterior faucial pillars. Dysphagia 2003;18:16–26.

7 Huckabee ML, Pelletier CA: Management of Adult Neurogenic Dysphagia. San Diego, Singular Publishing Group, 1999.

8 Gallas S, Marie JP, Leroi AM, Verin E: Sensory transcutaneous electrical stimulation improves post-stroke dysphagic patients. Dysphagia 2010;25:291–297.

9 Mistry S, Rothwell JC, Thompson DG, Hamdy S: Modulation of human cortical swallowing motor pathways after pleasant and aversive taste stimuli. Am J Physiol Gastrointest Liver Physiol 2006;291:G666–G671.

10 Theurer JA, Czachorowski KA, Martin LP, Martin RE: Effects of oropharyngeal air-pulse stimulation on swallowing in healthy older adults. Dysphagia 2009;24:302–313.

11 Soros P, Lalone E, Smith R, et al: Functional MRI of oropharyngeal air-pulse stimulation. Neuroscience 2008;153:1300–1308.

12 Teismann IK, Steinstrater O, Warnecke T, et al: Tactile thermal oral stimulation increases the cortical representation of swallowing. BMC Neurosci 2009;10:71.

13 Lowell SY, Poletto CJ, Knorr-Chung BR, et al: Sensory stimulation activates both motor and sensory components of the swallowing system. Neuroimage 2008;42:285–295.

14 Kahrilas PJ, Logemann JA, Gibbons P: Food intake by maneuver; an extreme compensation for impaired swallowing. Dysphagia 1992;7:155–159.

15 Kahrilas PJ, Logemann JA, Krugler C, Flanagan E: Volitional augmentation of upper esophageal sphincter opening during swallowing. Am J Physiol 1991;260:G450–G456.

16 Crary MA: A direct intervention program for chronic neurogenic dysphagia secondary to brainstem stroke. Dysphagia 1995;10:6–18.

17 Crary MA, Carnaby Mann GD, et al: Functional benefits of dysphagia therapy using adjunctive sEMG biofeedback. Dysphagia 2004;19:160–164.

18 Huckabee ML, Cannito M: Outcomes of swallowing rehabilitation in chronic brainstem dysphagia: a retrospective evaluation. Dysphagia 1999;14:93–109.

19 Burkhead LM, Sapienza CM, Rosenbek JC: Strength-training exercise in dysphagia rehabilitation: principles, procedures, and directions for future research. Dysphagia 2007;22:251–265.

20 Easterling C, Kern MK, Nitschke T, et al: Restoration of oral feeding in 17 tube fed patients by the Shaker Exercise. Dysphagia 2000;15:105.

21 Logemann JA, Rademaker A, Pauloski BR, et al: A randomized study comparing the Shaker exercise with traditional therapy: a preliminary study. Dysphagia 2009;24:403–411.

22 Sapienza CM: Respiratory muscle strength training applications. Curr Opin Otolaryngol Head Neck Surg 2008;16:216–220.

23 Wheeler-Hegland KM, Rosenbek JC, Sapienza CM: Submental sEMG and hyoid movement during Mendelsohn maneuver, effortful swallow, and expiratory muscle strength training. J Speech Lang Hear Res 2008;51:1072–1087.

24 Pitts T, Bolser D, Rosenbek J, Troche M, Okun MS, Sapienza C: Impact of expiratory muscle strength training on voluntary cough and swallow function in Parkinson disease. Chest 2009;135:1301–1308.

25 Troche MS, Okun MS, Rosenbek JC, et al: Aspiration and swallowing in Parkinson disease and rehabilitation with EMST: a randomized trial. Neurology 2010;75: 1912–1919.

26 Nicosia MA, Hind JA, Roecker EB, et al: Age effects on the temporal evolution of isometric and swallowing pressure. J Gerontol A Biol Sci Med Sci 2000;55:M634–M640.

27 Robbins J, Gangnon RE, Theis SM, et al: The effects of lingual exercise on swallowing in older adults. J Am Geriatr Soc 2005;53: 1483–1489.

28 Robbins J, Kays SA, Gangnon RE, et al: The effects of lingual exercise in stroke patients with dysphagia. Arch Phys Med Rehabil 2007;88:150–158.

29 Steele CM, Van Lieshout PHHM: Tongue movements during water swallowing in healthy younger and older adults. J Speech Lang Hear Res 2009;52:1255–1267.

30 Yeates EM, Molfenter SM, Steele CM: Improvements in tongue strength and pressure-generation precision following a tongue-pressure training protocol in older individuals with dysphagia: three case reports. Clin Interv Aging 2008;3:735–747.

Cichero J, Clavé P (eds): Stepping Stones to Living Well with Dysphagia.
Nestlé Nutr Inst Workshop Ser, vol 72, pp 119–126,
Nestec Ltd., Vevey/S. Karger AG., Basel, © 2012

Oropharyngeal Dysphagia Pathophysiology, Complications and Science-Based Interventions

Kenneth W. Altman

Mount Sinai School of Medicine, New York, NY, USA

Abstract

The etiology of oropharyngeal dysphagia can be broad, and includes aging with atrophy, debilitation, stroke, neurodegenerative and muscular diseases, tumor and postsurgical deformity, as well as effects due to medications and drying of the mucosal membranes. Pathophysiology depends on the multiple causative factors, including the cortex and neural connections to generate the swallow, as well as the oropharyngeal musculature. While chronic debilitation and age may result in nutritional deficiency and poor hydration, the other causes generally present with aspiration risk more acutely. Bacteriologically, aspiration pneumonia is usually polymicrobial with a predominance of Gram-negative enteric bacilli. However, there is emerging evidence to suggest that odontogenic sources may complicate the severity of bacterial load. The principles behind science-based interventions are primarily aspiration assessment with bedside evaluation, and ultimately modified barium swallow (videofluoroscopy) or functional endoscopic evaluation of swallowing (with or without sensory testing). Each has its advantages and logistical concerns. Intervention and rehabilitation is unique to the patient's needs, but may include reconditioning and therapy with a speech and language pathologist, and surgical options. The emerging roles of neuroplasticity and external neuromuscular stimulation are also discussed.

Introduction

Oropharyngeal dysphagia is impairment to a critical portion of the swallow mechanism. It results from a spectrum of associated diseases and disorders, as well as normal aging. While a normal intact swallow meets nutritional and hydration needs, oropharyngeal dysphagia chronically may result in malnutrition and dehydration. The oropharyngeal swallow involves a rapid, highly coordinated set of neuromuscular actions beginning with lip closure and terminating with opening of the upper esophageal sphincter [1]. Since the oropharyngeal component to swallowing is a critical portion that not only propels the bolus of food but also results in laryngeal protection, oropharyngeal dysphagia increases aspiration risk. This review paper is based on a series of presentations at the Second International Course on Oropharyngeal Dysphagia in Mataró Spain May 5–6, 2011, and the existing broad body of literature to supplement the subjects presented.

Pathophysiology of Oropharyngeal Dysphagia

The etiology of oropharyngeal dysphagia can be broad, and includes aging with atrophy, debilitation, stroke, neurodegenerative and muscular diseases, tumor and post-surgical deformity, as well as effects due to medications and drying of the mucosal membranes. Pathophysiology depends on the multiple causative factors, including the cortex and neural connections to generate the swallow, as well as the oropharyngeal musculature. The well-known phases of the swallow include oral preparatory, oral, oropharyngeal and esophageal. However, there is a strong suggestion to include cortical as well as laryngeal function.

Rofes et al. [2] explored the pathophysiology of oropharyngeal dysphagia in frail elderly patients (FEP), comparing 45 FEP (81.5 ± 1.1 years) with oropharyngeal dysphagia and 12 healthy volunteers (40 ± 2.4 years) via videofluoroscopy (VFS). Healthy volunteers demonstrated faster laryngeal closure, upper esophageal sphincter opening, maximal vertical hyoid motion, and stronger tongue propulsion forces. In the FEP group, 64% had oropharyngeal residue, 57% had laryngeal penetration and 17% had tracheobronchial aspiration. As expected, FEP with impaired swallow safety had higher 1-year mortality rates (51.7 vs. 13.3%, p = 0.021) than FEP with safe swallow. They concluded that weak tongue bolus propulsion forces, slow hyoid motion and delayed laryngeal ventricle closure result in the impaired efficacy and increased aspiration risk.

The cortical control of swallowing was recently reviewed by Michou and Hamdy [3]. They summarized the newer data from neurophysiologic and neuroimaging studies that emphasize the integration and interconnection of the diverse swallowing cortical network. It is also clear that sensory input influences swallowing cortical activation. As such, it may reasonably be suggested that cortical and brainstem function should be included as a critical component of the normal swallow, in addition to the oral, oropharyngeal and esophageal phases [4].

Table 1. Generation and pathophysiology of oropharyngeal dysphagia

Component of swallowing	Effect in disease
Cortex, brainstem	Direct effect from stroke Dementia Traumatic brain injury Neurodegenerative disease
Upper and lower motor neurons	Neurodegenerative disease Tumor or postsurgical
Tongue and pharynx muscles	Aging, deconditioning Neuromuscular degenerative disease Effects of sicca Tumor or postsurgical
Sensory receptors	Sensory defect from stroke Effects of sicca Tumor or postsurgical

With this in mind, the need for cognitive assessment in the bedside swallow study was addressed by Leder et al. [5] in an attempt to correlate the cognitive state with aspiration. They developed a protocol for dysphagia testing that began with verbal stimuli to determine patient orientation status and ability to follow single-step verbal commands including mouth opening, sticking out their tongue and smiling. They studied 4,070 patients over a 7-year period. They found the odds of liquid aspiration were 31% greater for patients not oriented to person, place, and time. Patients unable to follow single-step verbal commands were at 57% greater risk of aspirating liquids, 48% greater aspiration risk of aspirating puree consistency, and 69% at greater risk of being unsafe to take any oral intake.

Table 1 summarizes the physiologic components of a normal swallow required for intact oropharyngeal function. As demonstrated here, cortical awareness of the bolus in the mouth required to trigger the oropharyngeal phase can be affected by stroke, dementia, traumatic brain injury, and neurodegenerative disease (such as multiple sclerosis). Upper and lower motor neurons, also responsible for tongue thrust and pharyngeal squeeze in the oropharyngeal phase can similarly be affected by tumor or prior surgery of the neck or skull-base, as well as neurodegenerative disease (such as Parkinson's, and amyotrophic lateral sclerosis). Musculature necessary for the swallow is commonly affected by atrophy induced by aging, deconditioning and sarcopenia. Neuromuscular disease as in myasthenia gravis may also impair normal muscle function in the swallow. Sensation is supremely important to be able to recognize the bolus to have conscious and reflexive protective mechanisms against aspiration. Oral and laryngeal sicca also impair sensory function.

Complications of Oropharyngeal Dysphagia and Aspiration Bacteriology

While chronic debilitation and age may result in nutritional deficiency and poor hydration, the other causes generally present with aspiration risk more acutely. Bacteriologically, aspiration pneumonia is usually polymicrobial with a predominance of Gram-negative enteric bacilli. El-Solh et al. [6] investigated the microbial etiology and prognostic indicators of 95 institutionalized elders with severe aspiration pneumonia. Gram-negative enteric bacilli were the predominant organisms isolated (49%), followed by anaerobic bacteria (16%), and *Staphylococcus aureus* (12%), with a total of 67 pathogens identified. The crude mortality was 33% for the aerobic and 36% for the anaerobic group (p = 0.9), with hypoalbuminemia (p < 0.001) and the burden of comorbid diseases (p < 0.001) as independent risk factors of poor outcome.

Due to the presence of anaerobic bacteria in aspiration pneumonia, there is the suggestion that odontogenic sources may complicate the severity of bacterial load. This was addressed in a systematic review of 34 articles over a 40-year period [7]. The authors concluded that there was '(1) an association between poor oral hygiene and respiratory pathogens, (2) a decrease in the incidence of respiratory complications when patients are provided chemical or mechanical interventions for improved oral care, (3) the complex nature of periodontal disease and aspiration pneumonia make direct connections between the two challenging, and (4) additional studies are warranted to determine adequate oral hygiene protocols for nursing home patients to further reduce the incidence of aspiration pneumonia.'

Science-Based Assessment of Aspiration Risk

As discussed above, the bedside evaluation should always precede objective measurement of the swallowing mechanism and aspiration risk. In the compromised patient, all studies are dependent on patient performance and have the potential for precarious findings when a patient is fatigued. The main principles behind science-based assessment are primarily (1) identification of aspiration risk with bedside evaluation, and (2) ultimately modified barium swallow (VFS) or functional endoscopic evaluation of swallowing (FEES, with or without sensory testing). Each has its advantages and logistical concerns. Table 2 shows that VFS has the advantages over FEES of being able to examine the oral preparatory and oral phases, follow bolus during pharyngeal squeeze, and assess cricopharyngeal function and passage to esophagus. On the other hand, FEES has the unique advantages of being able to directly visualize nasopharyngeal and laryngeal anatomy, directly assess sensory defects, and possibly directly observe pooled secretions and aspiration of saliva before the swallow. There are also logistical concerns to be able to perform either test, as shown in table 3.

Table 2. Unique advantages of modified barium swallow (VFS) versus FEES

Modified barium swallow	FEES
Examines oral preparatory and oral phases	Directly visualize nasopharyngeal and laryngeal anatomy
Can follow bolus during pharyngeal squeeze	Can directly assess sensory defects
Assesses cricopharyngeal function and passage to esophagus	Directly observe pooled secretions and aspiration of saliva before the swallow

Table 3. Logistical concerns regarding modified barium swallow (VFS) versus FEES

Modified barium swallow	FEES
Exposure to radiation	No radiation
Requires speech pathologist, radiologist, and technician	Speech pathologist with or without otolaryngologist
Views real-time images (video), records still images	Records real-time images (for optimal reimbursement in USA), may show still images in report
Transport to radiology department	Performed at bedside or exam room

These include patient transport to a radiology department for VFS, exposure to radiation, and the need for multiple personnel such as the speech and language pathologist, radiologist and radiology technician. Many FEES systems also allow for the storage and retrieval of real-time images related to the swallow evaluation, whereas VFS usually views real-time images during the exam but saves static images for later retrieval and review. Ultimately, the test of choice depends on availability of resources and trained clinicians.

Tabaee et al. [8] compared the addition of sensory testing to FEES (FEESST) with VFS in dysphagia testing, reviewing 54 patients who underwent both studies within a 2-week period. Forty-one percent of patients were not eating by mouth at the time of FEESST, and the mean interval between the two examinations was 5 days. Laryngeal examination revealed edema/erythema in 93%, impaired pharyngeal squeeze in 66%, decreased laryngopharyngeal sensation in 82%, and absent laryngeal adductor reflex in 30%. FEESST with all consistencies revealed pooling in 89%, penetration in 83%, and aspiration in 65% of patients. VFS revealed pooling in 65%, penetration in 67%, and aspiration in 54% of patients. Comparison of FEESST and VFS revealed full agreement in 52%, minor disagreement in 13%, and major disagreement in 35% of patients.

The addition of fiberoptic endoscopic dysphagia severity scale (FEDSS) for acute stroke patients, grading dysphagia into 6 severity codes (1–6; 1 being best), has also been introduced [9]. Severity of FEDSS has been shown to be a predictor of functional outcome at 3 months after stroke, as measured by the modified Rankin Scale. Each increase of 1 point on the FEDSS conferred a more than 2-fold increased chance of developing pneumonia. The odds for the necessity of endotracheal intubation raised by a factor of nearly 2.5 with each additional point on the FEDSS.

Belafsky and Rees [10] later recognized the limitation of FEES not exploring the esophagus for a comprehensive assessment of dysphagia, and compared 21 patients who had guided observation of esophageal swallowing with concurrent VFS and/or manometry. They found concurrence in 71% with VFS, and 83% with manometry. More importantly, the procedure identified pathology not detected by fluoroscopy and manometry in 62% of patients.

Science-Based Interventions and Discussion

Intervention and rehabilitation is unique to the patient's needs, but may include reconditioning and therapy with a speech and language pathologist, and surgical options. Ashford et al. [11] performed a systematic review of behavioral interventions for dysphagia, predominantly of neurological origin (brain injury, stroke, Parkinson's disease, and dementia). The seven behavioral treatments investigated included three postural interventions (side lying, chin tuck, and head rotation) and four swallowing maneuvers (effortful swallow, Mendelsohn, supraglottic swallow, and super-supraglottic swallow). While many of these are used in clinical practice, the authors found a paucity of objective evidence in the literature, and no studies were found to address the effortful swallow or the super-supraglottic swallow.

There are, however, emerging potential roles for the concept of neuroplasticity in therapy, and for transcutaneous electrical stimulation (TES) in selected cases. In a working group of experts in swallowing and dysphagia, 10 principles of neural plasticity were proposed that suggested the potential for therapeutic interventions that can change targeted physiology related to dysphagia [12]. One example may be the use of alternative sensory pathways as feedback during the swallow in a patient with partially impaired laryngeal sensation. Muscular plasticity should also be of benefit not only through reconditioning the atrophic muscles, but also in the way of using novel muscle groups to compensate for permanent impairments in other muscle groups needed for functional swallowing. While there is little objective evidence suggesting the role of neuroplasticity for dysphagia interventions thus far, there appears to be enough analogous evidence to suggest its potential.

There is still controversy surrounding the use of TES on the neck for dysphagia rehabilitation. The target of stimulation is commonly the hyolaryngeal complex which is needed for laryngeal elevation, and thus laryngeal protection during the oropharyngeal swallow. While studies demonstrate hyolaryngeal depression when the lower neck is stimulated, submental TES has not been found to effectively elevate the hyolaryngeal complex [13]. However, further study in this and other emerging technologies is warranted.

Conclusion

This review focuses on the pathophysiology of oropharyngeal dysphagia, particularly as it relates to cortical dysfunction in a variety of disease states and aging. Clinical assessment when a patient presents with signs of aspiration or aspiration pneumonia requires bedside and objective assessment, including FEES, FEESST and VFS. Behavioral interventions are frequently used in oropharyngeal dysphagia rehabilitation, yet there is a paucity of evidence and further study is warranted. The emerging concept of therapy target at neuroplasticity as well as other proposed technologies offers encouraging options on the horizon for the treatment of oropharyngeal dysphagia.

References

1 Logemann JA, Larsen K: Oropharyngeal dysphagia: pathophysiology and diagnosis for the anniversary issue of *Diseases of the Esophagus*. Dis Esophagus 2011;25:299–304.
2 Rofes L, Arreola V, Romea M, et al: Pathophysiology of oropharyngeal dysphagia in the frail elderly. Neurogastroenterol Motil 2010;22:851–858.
3 Michou E, Hamdy S: Cortical input in control of swallowing. Curr Opin Otolaryngol Head Neck Surg 2009;17:166–171.
4 Altman KW: Dysphagia evaluation and care in the hospital setting: the need for protocolization. Otolaryngol Head Neck Surg 2011;145:895–898.
5 Leder SB, Suiter DM, Lisitano Warner H: Answering orientation questions and following single-step verbal commands: effect on aspiration status. Dysphagia 2009;24:290–295.
6 El-Solh AA, Pietrantoni C, Bhat A, et al: Microbiology of severe aspiration pneumonia in institutionalized elderly. Am J Respir Crit Care Med 2003;167:1650–1654.
7 Pace CC, McCullough GH: The association between oral microorgansims and aspiration pneumonia in the institutionalized elderly: review and recommendations. Dysphagia 2010;25:307–322.
8 Tabaee A, Johnson PE, Gartner CJ, et al: Patient-controlled comparison of flexible endoscopic evaluation of swallowing with sensory testing (FEESST) and videofluoroscopy. Laryngoscope 2006;116:821–825.
9 Warnecke T, Ritter MA, Kroger B, et al: Fiberoptic endoscopic dysphagia severity scale predicts outcome after acute stroke. Cerebrovasc Dis 2009;28:283–289.
10 Belafsky PC, Rees CJ: Functional oesophagoscopy: endoscopic evaluation of the oesophageal phase of deglutition. J Laryngol Otol 2009;123:1031–1034.

11 Ashford J, McCabe D, Wheeler-Hegland K, et al: Evidence-based systematic review: oropharyngeal dysphagia behavioral treatments. III. Impact of dysphagia treatments on populations with neurological disorders. J Rehabil Res Dev 2009;46:195–204.

12 Robbins J, Butler SG, Daniels SK, et al: Swallowing and dysphagia rehabilitation: translating principles of neural plasticity into clinically oriented evidence. J Speech Lang Hear Res 2008;51:S276–S300.

13 Ludlow CL: Electrical neuromuscular stimulation in dysphagia: current status. Curr Opin Otolaryngol Head Neck Surg 2010;18:159–164.

Cichero J, Clavé P (eds): Stepping Stones to Living Well with Dysphagia.
Nestlé Nutr Inst Workshop Ser, vol 72, pp 127–133,
Nestec Ltd., Vevey/S. Karger AG., Basel, © 2012

Concluding Remarks

Our first aim is to acknowledge the faculty and the speakers for their contribution and preparation of the articles, presentations and materials for the course 72nd Nestlé Nutrition Institute Workshop 'Stepping Stones to Living Well with Dysphagia' and also to acknowledge the attendees for the high level of interaction and discussion. The first – 2010 – edition of this course was inaugurated by *Michel Gardet*, CEO of Nestlé Healthcare Nutrition, and the second – 2011 – by *Petra Klassen*, Medical and Scientific Affairs Manager at Nestlé, showing the high relevance of the topic dysphagia for the Nestlé Nutrition Institute mission of sharing science-based information and education on Nutrition. The venue for the 2010 and 2011 workshops was the Hospital de Mataró in Barcelona, Spain. These concluding remarks summarize the rich information surrounding oropharyngeal dysphagia that was presented and discussed during the 2010 and 2011 Workshops and have been included in this book.

The first session of the 2011 Workshop started with the discussion on the prevalence of oropharyngeal dysphagia with *Julie Cichero*, and the consequences of dysphagia on prognosis of patients and hospital resources with *Kenneth Altman*. These initial presentations are summarized in the first chapter of this book 'Definition, prevalence, and burden of oropharyngeal dysphagia: a serious problem among older adults worldwide and the impact on prognosis and hospital resources' by these authors. This chapter describes the true prevalence of dysphagia is difficult to determine as it has been reported as a function of care setting, disease state and country of investigation. However, extrapolating from the literature, in older adults, oropharyngeal dysphagia presents with a prevalence of 11% in the community, more than 25% in acute hospitals and upwards of 55% in aged care settings. Consequences of dysphagia include malnutrition, dehydration, aspiration pneumonia and potentially death. The mean cost for an aspiration pneumonia episode of care is USD 17,000, rising with the number of comorbid conditions. Whilst financial costs can be objectively counted, the despair, depression, and social isolation are more difficult to quantify. *Kenneth Altman* argued that dysphagia is an underrecognized condition that contributes to a 40% increased length of stay and 13-fold increased mortality during hospitalization for elderly patients. Both sufferers and their families bear the social and psychological burden of dysphagia. There may be a cost-effective role for screening and early identification of dysphagia, particularly in high-risk populations. During the discussion, *Pere Clavé* pointed out that the World Health Organization has recently established a specific code for oropharyngeal dysphagia within its International Classification of Diseases (ICD-10) system (http://www.who.int/classifications/icd/en). He acknowledged that dysphagia has not traditionally been considered a disease, but rather a symptom or component of many other disease and injury conditions, but argued that our understanding and appreciation of dysphagia prevalence and epidemiology would be significantly advanced if initiatives were taken to encourage physicians to use the oropharyngeal dysphagia code in their medical reports. *Pere Clavé* mentioned that the European Society for Swallowing Disorders would be launching an initiative along these lines called 'Dysphagia Day' in cooperation with the Dysphagia Research Society – represented by *Rosemary Martino* during the discussions – and interested clinicians from South America – *Roberto Dantas*, and Japan. Another audience member, *Carola Granholm*, pointed out that similar concerns have been raised regarding the recognition and awareness of malnutrition in the elderly, and that the ESPEN, the European Society for Parenteral and Enteral Nutrition has been working for several years to improve awareness about malnutrition in the EU. She argued that awareness may need to be raised to the political level if the necessary financial resources are going to be made available to properly address the burden of dysphagia for our aging population. *Michael Jedwab* proposed that early identification and diagnosis would serve to stop the negative cycle of malnutrition and pneumonia risk that seems to spiral out of control when dysphagia is not recognized. The remaining talks in the opening session of the conference addressed the specifics of the pathophysiology of dysphagia and aspiration. *Shaheen Hamdy* reviewed the neurophysiology of swallowing, and described methods for mapping the swallowing neural pathways, both sensory and motor, that are used in his laboratory. *Pere Clavé* described issues related to the timing of the swallow response and the reconfiguration of the oropharynx from a respiratory passage to an alimentary passage. *Julie Cichero* along with *Eric Verin* discussed issues of respiratory-swallow coordination. The main concepts described in these presentations and the pathophysiology and complications of oropharyngeal dysphagia were discussed by *Catriona Steele*.

The second session of the Workshop was dedicated to screening and clinical assessment of oropharyngeal dysphagia, with *Kala Kaspar* presenting the 10-item Eating Assessment Tool (EAT-10), *Viridiana Arreola* presenting the volume-viscosity test for dysphagia and aspiration (V-VST), *Renée Speyer* reviewing the effectiveness and feasibility of bedside methods for detecting oropharyngeal dysphagia, and *Rosemary Martino* leading the discussion of all these topics on screening and bedside clinical diagnosis. This book contains a chapter detailing how to identify vulnerable patients and the role of the EAT-10 and the multidisciplinary team in early intervention and comprehensive dysphagia care by *Kala Kaspar* and *Olle Ekberg*. It shows systematic screening with a validated method (e.g. EAT-10) as part of a comprehensive care protocol enables multidisciplinary teams to more effectively manage the condition, reduce the economic and societal burden, and improve patient quality of life. Screening for dysphagia allows individuals to be quickly and accurately identified for formal swallowing assessment and intervention. The EAT-10 is a validated tool that is broadly applicable to individuals with dysphagia. Both patients and clinicians can use the EAT-10 to identify dysphagia risk. Following identification of oropharyngeal dysphagia using a validated screening tool, formal assessment of dysphagia is required. Tools such as the V-VST have been shown to provide valuable information regarding the need for instrumental assessment of swallowing (e.g. videofluoroscopy, VFS, or endoscopy). In an independent chapter, *Viridiana Arreola* on behalf of the Mataró team described the V-VST for bedside clinical assessment of dysphagia and aspiration. Oropharyngeal dysphagia can affect swallowing safety, resulting in potential aspiration or pneumonia. It can also affect efficiency of swallowing, resulting in potential malnutrition and dehydration. The V-VST affords accurate clinical assessment of both safety and efficiency and also the most appropriate bolus volume and viscosity for each patient. The V-VST identifies patients who need further exploration by VFS and helps to select the ideal bolus volume and viscosity for liquids when a VFS study cannot be performed. Development of the V-VST (long-form) now includes two additional thickness levels, allowing for more precise allocation of fluid thickness required for individual patient safety. The V-VST can be administered by any member of the multidisciplinary dysphagia team, facilitating the clinical assessment of dysphagia at all medical facilities and at any time of day, and can be repeated according the natural progression of the disease. *Patricia Anthony* led a relevant discussion on the difference between methods for clinical screening of dysphagia – fast and simple methods aimed to select patients with symptoms at risk for the condition – and clinical assessment methods – more formal, and accurate methods of clinical exploration aimed to provide a formal diagnosis of oropharyngeal dysphagia and guide those patients needing complementary explorations. Following these discussions, a practical session on bedside clinical assessment using the V-VST ensued. Participants were divided into groups of ~20 on the 2nd Floor of Hospital de Mataró (Medicine, Geriatrics, Neurology wards), and V-VST examinations were performed on real patients by the team of nurses with *Rosa Monteis*, *Anna Ciurana*, *Marisa Sebastian* and *Viridiana Arreola*.

Session 3 on day 1 was dedicated to instrumental diagnosis and complementary explorations in the patient with oropharyngeal dysphagia with talks on the videofluoroscopic swallow study by *Margareta Bülow*, fiberoptic endoscopic evaluation of swallowing (FEES): techniques, signs, and reports with examples in head and neck cancer patients by *Daniele Farneti*, and the evolution of the diagnostic strategies for oropharyngeal dysphagia by *Roberto Dantas*. Instrumental assessment of swallowing function allows the clinician to determine the exact cause of the swallowing dysfunction in order to better plan treatment. In addition, instrumental examination is able to disclose silent aspiration. Disorders of timing, coordination, and degree of impairment can be identified. The use of different food textures and liquid viscosities, in addition to swallowing maneuvers allows the clinician to prescribe the best course of treatment for each individual. The benefits of multidisciplinary teamwork are also conveyed in the chapter 'Therapeutic Videoradiographic Swallowing Study' where *Margareta Bülow* writes that the combined skills of a speech language pathologist and radiologist are utilized to identify the main VFS signs of dysphagia. Different textures as well as different therapeutic strategies can be tested during the examination. Any swallowing dysfunction shows individual characterization, and therefore recommendations regarding safe and efficient nutrition, have to be based on the individuals' actual pathophysiology. Either modified textures or if necessary tube feeding and/or different therapeutic strategies could be prescribed. This session ended with a constructive discussion on the complementary diagnostic role of VFS and FEES. Where endoscopy is used as the instrumental medium, the nasopharyngeal and laryngeal mucosa, and secretions in the pharynx and around the larynx can be visualized and any anatomical-structural alteration assessed. Some endoscopy instruments allow for testing of sensory function, providing welcome additional information. In an additional practical session 2 on how to measure the swallow response by the videofluoroscopic swallow study, clinical examples by *Margareta Bülow* and *Pere Clavé* allowed the participants to discuss real examples of the main VFS signs and their clinical relevance.

Day 1 of the workshop finished with a session dedicated to reviewing the pathophysiology, relevance and natural history of oropharyngeal dysphagia among patient groups including neurogenic dysphagia by *Ernest Palomeras*, elderly by *Pere Clavé*, and aspiration pneumonia: a life-threatening complication of oropharyngeal dysphagia and the need for comprehensive care by a multidisciplinary team by *Jordi Almirall*. This book contains two chapters dedicated to the elderly and to aspiration pneumonia. The first one is dedicated to the pathophysiology, relevance and natural history of oropharyngeal dysphagia among older people and describes the relationship between oropharyngeal dysphagia, sarcopenia and the impaired neural elements of swallow response in older persons, with prolonged and delayed laryngeal vestibule closure and slow hyoid movement causing oropharyngeal aspirations. Oropharyngeal dysphagia causes malnutrition, dehydration, impaired quality of life, lower respiratory tract infections, aspiration pneumonia, and poor prognosis including prolonged hospital stay and enhanced morbidity and mortality in several phenotypes of older patients ranging from independently living older people, hospitalized older patients and nursing home residents. We discussed that oropharyngeal dysphagia should be recognized as a major geriatric syndrome, and we recommend a policy of systematic and universal screening and assessment of oropharyngeal dysphagia among older people to prevent its severe complications. In his chapter, *Jordi Almirall* writes that patients who aspirate may or may not go on to develop the life threatening condition of aspiration pneumonia. Exact prevalence figures for aspiration pneumonia are difficult to determine from the literature. It is clear that prevalence resulting in hospitalization increases with advancing age and that neurodegenerative conditions and stroke significantly increase risk for the development of aspiration pneumonia. Frail elderly and nursing home residents have a 10-fold increased risk of developing aspiration pneumonia. It is the third highest cause of mortality in individuals over 85 years of age. The pathogenesis of aspiration pneumonia depends on two elements: (a) factors affecting oropharyngeal or gastroesophageal motility, and (b) factors favoring bacterial colonization of oropharyngeal or gastrointestinal secretions. Although there is a high preponderance of Gram-negative enteric bacilli load, dental sources of bacteria most likely also impact the severity of the bacterial load. Risk factors for the development of aspiration pneumonia relating to advancing age, poor dental hygiene, malnutrition, current history of smoking, use of aerosol inhalers, dehydration, intubation and a weakened immune system have been identified. It is worth bearing in mind the relative unimportance of anaerobic bacteria in aspiration pneumonia. Treatment aimed at reducing these risk factors, and the most appropriate antibiotic treatments were also discussed.

We started Day 2 with a discussion of the nutritional complications of dysphagia, the screening and assessment of nutritional status with *Patricia Anthony*, treatment of malnutrition and sarcopenia with *Rosa Burgos*, dietary modifications by *Didier Bleeckx*, nutritional support by *Alfonso Cruz Jenthoft*, and a discussion on this led by *Juan Ochoa*. Malnutrition and dehydration remain large-scale complications for individuals with oropharyngeal dysphagia. Like the need to identify individuals at risk of dysphagia, there is an equally important need to identify the risk for malnutrition. The global prevalence of malnutrition is upwards of 22%, increasing in hospital and rehabilitation settings. Tools such as the Malnutrition Screening Assessment-Short Form offer an expedient, validated and reliable tool for just such a purpose. Malnutrition contributes to reduction in muscle mass and strength (sarcopenia). These factors increase the risk of falls and fractures as seen in deterioration of large muscles, and may contribute directly to oropharyngeal dysphagia with deterioration of the smaller muscles used for swallowing. An increase in the level of disability and a reduction in independence are further consequences. The risk of sarcopenia increases with typical aging. Evidence-based treatment to manage sarcopenia includes resistance exercises, with or without nutritional supplementation. In addition to sarcopenia, malnutrition contributes to inadequacies of the immune system and subsequent deficiencies in wound healing. Nutritional counseling needs to be considered as good practice in proactive management of elderly individuals. A good nutritional status improves quality of life, life expectancy and reduces disability. Nutritional needs change along the course of a lifetime. Clinicians need to be cognizant that the nutritional needs of the elderly are different to those of younger adults. Due to the numerous conditions associated with aging (cardiovascular disease, neurological impairment, etc.) and coexisting medical conditions, there is a further need to individualize nutritional counseling for the elderly.

In order to meet the nutritional needs of individuals with dysphagia, food textures may be altered and liquids thickened. Individuals may also benefit from oral supplementation to ensure they are receiving their required daily intake levels. For some individuals, dietary needs may only be met by supplementation (nasogastric or enteric tube). Individuals with dysphagia have more than double the risk for developing malnutrition than those individuals without dysphagia. The adequate identification and management of *dysphagia and malnutrition* require the skills of a multidisciplinary team. Health professionals need to be familiar with the risk factors for *both* conditions and identify pathways for referral of patients for optimum care. Nutrition intervention needs to commence early for the hospitalized patient. Frequent reviews of both swallowing function and nutrition are required as the patient moves through the health care system in order for optimal care to occur. All these nutritional issues related to oropharyngeal dysphagia are summarized in this book in three important chapters: one by *Rosa Burgos*, discussing the therapeutic approach to malnutrition and sarcopenia, one by *Alfonso Cruz-Jenthof*, discussing the importance of nutritional support in older people, and a chapter from *Juan Ochoa*, discussing nutrition assessment and intervention in the patient with dysphagia and the challenges for quality improvement.

Part 2 of Day 2 was dedicated to treatment of oropharyngeal dysphagia. First a practical session led by *Mireia Arús* and *Maria Roca* was on how to assure safe and appealing nutrition for optimal compliance and outcomes, and provided the participants with the opportunity to use the commercial thickening agents available worldwide to prepare thickened liquids according to a particular clinical situation. A block was dedicated to treatment with swallow rehabilitation and oral health dealing with swallow rehabilitation by *Catriona Steele*, the potential pharmacological approach by *Laia Rofes*, oral health issues by *José Nart*. A discussion led by *Rosemary Martino* was used to describe the available and future methods of treatment. This book contains a chapter from *Kenneth Altman* reviewing oropharyngeal dysphagia pathophysiology, complications and science-based interventions. He describes behavioral interventions that are frequently used in oropharyngeal dysphagia rehabilitation, yet there is a paucity of evidence, and further study is warranted. The emerging concept of therapeutic targets of neuroplasticity, as well as other proposed technologies offers encouraging options on the horizon for the treatment of oropharyngeal dysphagia.

Finally a chapter on rehabilitative techniques for dysphagia by *Catriona Steele* describes three promising rehabilitation techniques for improving muscle strength and function related to swallowing: the Shaker exercise, expiratory muscle strength training, and tongue pressure resistance training. All three techniques invoke principles of task specificity, muscular load, resistance, and intensity, and aim to achieve functional changes in swallowing through changes in muscle physiology derived from strength or endurance training. To date, studies of treatment benefit arising from these techniques involve small sample sizes; this is particularly true of randomized studies with controls receiving standard treatment or experiencing spontaneous recovery. Nevertheless, a review of the available literature shows that improvement of penetration-aspiration is a common finding for individuals with dysphagia receiving one of these three treatment approaches. Although hypothesized as an expected outcome of swallow muscle strength training, improvements in post-swallow residues are noted to be uncommon as an outcome of these exercise-based approaches. The available evidence suggests that exercise-based approaches to swallowing rehabilitation do succeed in changing muscle strength and function, but generalization to true swallowing tasks may be somewhat limited.

In summary, the main conclusion of the 72nd Nestlé Nutrition Institute Workshop 'Stepping Stones to Living Well with Dysphagia' is that oropharyngeal dysphagia is a very prevalent disease resulting in life-changing events related to the everyday requirements for eating and drinking. Some of these events, i.e. dehydration, malnutrition, and pneumonia, are life-threatening. There is under-recognition of the prevalence of oropharyngeal dysphagia and little awareness that the condition can be identified by screening, and treated and managed by the combined skills of a multidisciplinary team. The physical, psychological, financial and social burden of oropharyngeal dysphagia impacts on the patients, their carers, and the health system that supports them. Clinicians are encouraged to use screening and assessment methods and internationally recognized codes such as the ICD-10 to identify dysphagia in order that this condition receives the attention it requires.

We also want to acknowledge the excellent organization led by *Andreas Bush* from Nestlé Healthcare Nutrition, *Susana Sancelestino* from the Yellow agency and her team for developing the webinars, the cooperation of all our patients and the hospitality of the Healthcare Team at the venue of the Hospital de Mataró, Consorci Sanitari del Maresme, Spain.

Julie Cichero
Pere Clavé

Subject Index

β-Adrenergic agonists, sarcopenia
    management 98
Aging, *see* Elderly
American College of Chest Physicians
    (ACCP), dysphagia screening
    guidelines 21–24, 27
Androstenedione, sarcopenia
    management 90
Angiotensin-converting enzyme (ACE),
    sarcopenia management with
    inhibitors 97, 98
Aspiration, risk assessment in
    oropharyngeal dysphagia 27–29
Aspiration pneumonia (AP)
    antibiotic therapy 72
    definition 67, 68
    economic burden 127
    frequency 68
    microbiology 71, 72, 122
    prevention 72–74
    risk factors
        age 68, 70
        antibiotics 70
        dehydration 70
        dental hygiene 68, 69
        gastric pH increase 70, 71
        inhalers and aerosols 70
        malnutrition 69
        nasogastric tubes and
            intubation 70, 71
        smoking 69, 70
    risks with dysphagia and
        assessment 54, 122–124

Beta-agonists, *see* β-Adrenergic agonists

Complications, *see specific complications*
Costs, *see* Economic burden

Deglutition
    definition 2
    pathophysiology of oropharyngeal
        dysphagia 120, 121
    physiology 54
Dehydroepiandrosterone (DHEA),
    sarcopenia management 89, 90
Dysphagia
    definition 2
    oropharyngeal versus esophageal 2, 3
Dysphagia Day 128

Eating Assessment Tool (EAT-10),
    dysphagia screening and
    monitoring 24–27, 29, 128, 129
Economic burden, oropharyngeal
    dysphagia 6–9, 15
Elderly, oropharyngeal dysphagia
    complications 62, 63
    malnutrition, *see* Malnutrition
    muscle loss, *see* Sarcopenia
    natural history 61–63
    pathophysiology 58–61
    prevalence 58
    prognosis 63
    treatment 64, 65
Estrogen replacement therapy, sarcopenia
    management 90, 91